Overcoming ADHD Without Medication

A Guidebook for Parents and Teachers

Overcoming ADHD Without Medication
A Guidebook for Parents and Teachers

Attention Deficit Hyperactivity Disorder (ADHD)
is a battle that can be won…
…….without the need for medication

The Association for Youth, Children
and Natural Psychology

NorthEast Books and Publishing
Newark, NJ

Overcoming
ADHD without Medication
A Guidebook for Parents and Teachers

English

Printed in the USA
NorthEast Books & Publishing
Newark, NJ

ISBN-10 982992432
ISBN-13 978-0-9829924-3-2
Library of Congress Control No. 201193904

All correspondence: editor@northeastbookspublishing.net

Photos on cover or elsewhere in this book, or quotes and articles from authors, authorities or other sources do not necessarily signify an endorsement of the views expressed in this book, unless otherwise stated.

All photos are for illustrative purposes only. Images are from paid photographers or services with professional models. There is no real-life connection between models of adults or children in this book, and the theme of the book, or the subject being illustrated.

Cover Photos -istockphoto.com **-** left to right
photographers: 1. Plainview 2. stock photo 3. STUDIO1ONE/Miroslav Ferkuniak 4. mammamaart
5. Stalman 6. absolute-india 7. stock photo 8. Abejon Photography 9. kzenon
10. bonniej graphic design

This book is dedicated to the children of Paterson, Newark, Elizabeth and Jersey City, NJ

Acknowledgements

Special thanks to Joel Nigg from Michigan State University, for his inspiring work and personal help. Thanks to Carol Confher for her support and insight from years of working with special education children. Thanks, also, to Jackie McGraw, from Paterson, NJ public library for her work with children, and who was one of the initial sources of inspiration for the research that went into this book. Also, thanks to Russell Barkley for his help and guidance in the initial stages of research. Thanks to J.W. for his help with editing and M.W. for her support and insight. Thanks also to school psychologist Keisha Hill for her support, insight, and statements, as well as to Kim Booker, Paterson, NJ grade school teacher, for her passionate dedication to help her students. Also, special thanks to Daniella Barroqueira of Illinois State University for providing her personal experience with ADHD, and to art teacher Ryan M. of Newark Public Schools for allowing us to reprint his inspiring experience. Thanks also to David Rabiner of Duke University for his valuable life-work with ADHD research and children's mental health, and for his permission to reprint samples of his insightful work on ADHD and depression. Also, thanks to Iowa State Public Relations and to the Iowa State University researchers for making their valuable research available to the public, and for reprint in this publication. Also, thanks to Sandra Rief for her excellent work for teachers as well as Dianne Levin. There are others not named here, including school psychologist, social workers, special education teachers and principals whose positive approach, encouragement, and skill in leading their schools, also provided examples used in this book.

Important Note – Please Read

The information presented in this book is intended for informative and educational purposes and not as a medical directive. The *AYCNP* is headed by educators and educational professionals, (rather than by psychologists or medical professionals), with a background in science and health education as well as certification in teaching psychology, and educational leadership, although much of the information in this book was derived from the work of psychologists and other professionals. By reading this publication the reader acknowledges that he or she maintains full responsibility in treatment choices for him or herself or for one's children or children under one's care.

This book does not replace professional treatment if necessary, but rather, complements it. By reading this book, the reader acknowledges his or her own freedom of choice in seeking medical treatment, and agrees that the *Association for Youth, Children and Natural Psychology*, as well as any individuals associated with the *Association for Youth, Children and Natural Psychology*, including authors quoted in this book, bear no responsibility for one's own personal choices in mental health, or other medical treatment, for him or herself or for one's children.

Readers are encouraged to gather as much information as possible from a variety of reliable sources when making medical choices involving mental health, evaluate the options, and make informed and balanced decisions.

Anyone who personally experiences suicidal thoughts, or anyone whose children are experiencing suicidal thoughts, should seek support from qualified professionals.

Preface

Ryan is an art teacher in a grade and middle school in Newark, NJ. He is well-liked by students and staff, is a great and productive artist, both in school and at home, and his students enjoy his class. When Ryan was in middle school and high school, he was diagnosed with ADHD, and was on stimulant medicines during those years. He says that he strongly disliked taking the medication, it made him feel "not himself," and one of the side effects of the stimulants for him was anger. When he got into college, he quit taking stimulants, but what helped him was being thoroughly immersed in artwork, he was an art major. Art helped him to focus. Playing soccer regularly helped his hyperactivity, and he never went back on medicine. No one today would have any reason to guess that he ever had problems associated with ADHD. (You can read a more detailed experience of Ryan on page 81). (You can read a more detailed experience of Ryan on page 81). Ryan's experience is not unique, and bits and pieces of his experience show up in the stories of many children and teens with ADHD.

Most parents are reluctant for their children to take stimulant medication, many are concerned with the side effects of ADHD medication, usually stimulants such as methylphenidate, most commonly referred to as Ritalin, and amphetamines, prescribed under various names. (Ritalin is not a true amphetamine, but is similar to an amphetamine). Many parents also question what the long-term effects might be for a child or teen taking stimulant medicines for years.

This book was produced while working with many children and teens with ADHD, through research, and through summarizing the work and ideas of many professionals in the field. The basis for the book ommenced in 2005, and reflects the lifework of dedicated professionals. It endeavors to present the information in a simple, concise form that is easily assimilated by busy parents and teachers, so that children might have a fuller opportunity for a ADHD symptom-free childhood through their teenage years.

A reading coach at a public library in Paterson, NJ, described her work with children, and how through help from supportive professionals, and with some simple lifestyle changes, such as attention to diet and nutrition, along with attentive support from parents, many children who were labeled as ADHD, were helped to cope with and to overcome symptoms of the disorder.

Russell Barkley is a well known author on the subject of ADHD, and his personal communication, as well as his encouragement to read Joel Nigg's then soon-to-be-released book, 2006, *What Causes ADHD?, Understanding What Goes Wrong and Why*, added further fuel to the research found here.

As it turns out, there is no single answer to the question, "What causes ADHD?," and there is no single child or teen whose genetic makeup or situation is exactly the same, so there is no single solution to the problem of overcoming ADHD.

There are certain principles of mental health and health which apply across the board, and there are certain logical observations which have been scientifically corroborated since the time that the research for this book began.

It seemed too much of a coincidence that in the same school district where many children played five hours of video games a day, which is certainly not unique to any geographic region in the United States or the world, that there would be, what was described by one school psychologist, an "epidemic" of cases of ADHD. A pre-teen boy who was labeled ADHD, and who began taking stimulant medications, also played around five hours of video games daily during the school week, in addition to watching movies and television on the weekends. The boy was on a high-sugar diet, and being raised by a single parent.

Clinical studies indicate that watching too much television as a child, might contribute to later symptoms of ADHD. Further, clinical studies provide a definite link between playing violent video games and with both aggression, and symptoms associated with ADHD. Given that the majority of children and teens today in the inner cities are either playing violent video games or watching violent movies from a young age (evidence for that is presented later in this book), it seems to be a reasonable conclusion that this might be affecting the mental health of many. Media is just one issue that parents should consider when addressing the topic of ADHD.

There are many positive lifestyle adjustments that can help children and teens who manifest symptoms of ADHD. Additionally, with any mental health difficulty or disorder, developing a personal list or arsenal of coping skills helps any individual to cope and even overcome symptoms associated with that disorder.

Yes, ADHD is being over-diagnosed today, according to what seems to be the most accurate research, and yes, medication for ADHD is over-prescribed. Parents, then, need to carefully consider their choices in this regard. There is much evidence that a child and teen can overcome ADHD without medication, which in the long-term, for most children, is a better option than taking stimulant drugs.

There is certainly a genetic component for children who develop symptoms of ADHD. Why does one child in the same family, living in the same environment, develop ADHD and the other two in the same basic age group don't?

However, like any mental health disorder, ADHD is not pure

genetics. It is more than likely a combination of genetics, environmental factors and social stressors. Many of these factors can be deliberately changed and modified, and making lifestyle changes can help many children overcome ADHD symptoms. Parents should consider what changes they can make in their lifestyle, what new coping skills their child can learn and develop. They may be amazed at the positive results with their child.

This book is not intended as a rule book for parents, and it is not assumed to be the final word or ultimate guide on the subject. There are many sources that you can turn to, especially in the past three or four years, which provide insightful ideas on self-help for ADHD. This is one source that will hopefully help many families, but that might also be a springboard for further investigation in the future.

Additionally, this book is not relating or documenting the experiences of one individual, rather, it represents the combined life-work of many dedicated individuals who work with children daily, and of others who have made it their life's work to research serious children's issues. It offers a cross-section of information from many sources on what can help children, parents and teachers, in addition to the experiences of those who have put this work together.

We wish you success in helping your child to overcome symptoms of ADHD, and hope that this book helps you along in your understanding of the disorder, as well as in developing coping skills and implementing lifestyle changes, which can help your child to overcome ADHD without medication.

****

The Association for Youth, Children and Natural Psychology (AYCNP) is a registered New Jersey non-profit corporation since 2008. Part of the proceeds from this publication are filtered back to the community for various modest endeavors towards the development and benefit of children and youth, as well as towards mental health education, non-pharmaceutical treatment, self-help, and prevention.

Kindly contact the AYCNP at aycnp@winmentalhealth.com for any suggestions for future editions of this book. Thank you.

Contents

"Masking the symptoms rather than removing the cause of the problems has always retarded the development of community health. The most fruitful area of research would be in prevention." Lawrence Green, Ph.D., J.M. Ottoson, Ph.D., 1999. *Community Population and Health.*

Introduction

A reading coach from the Paterson, NJ public library spoke firsthand about her experiences with children with ADHD. She had worked with hundreds of children who had been diagnosed with ADHD, or who were on the borderline of being classified, and she felt that the vast majority of these children could be helped, if their parents were given support and educated on how to help their children, through positive changes in the child's diet, as well as with support from services such as provided by the library program. The Paterson public library provided services for individual attention in reading to children, after school.

She explained that in all her years of professional work, having personally worked with hundreds of such children, she had only encountered a handful who she felt truly qualified as having ADHD. In those cases, none of these students had gone on medication, and were helped without medication through non-pharmaceutical professional support and simple lifestyle changes that parents were encouraged to implement, as well as through extra time and attention from concerned and supportive parents.

Art seems to have a positive affect for children who are diagnosed with ADHD. The quiet, solitude, and positive peaceful stimuli, helps children to focus. Supplementary material from Illinois State professor Daniella Barroqueira, Ph.D., who herself has ADHD, and whose experience is mirrored by a Newark grade school art teacher referred to in this book, helps to support the view that art can help some children, youth and adults, to cope with and overcome symptoms of ADHD, that some children and youth with ADHD are highly-visual and creative, and that the negative of ADHD can be turned into a positive.

A grade school art teacher and colleague who had been labeled as ADHD and who took Ritalin, and later Adderall, through middle school and high school years, explained that what he disliked the most about it was "the label". It made him feel different, set apart from the other kids. (When a child feels social stigma from a psychiatric label such as ADHD, this can be even more detrimental in the long-term than the symptoms associated with the disorder itself. See David Rabiner, page 89). When he was on the stimulants, he never felt himself, and the medicine contributed to anger problems. He said that what did help, was when he went to college, immersing himself in art and playing soccer. The art helped him to focus and the soccer was just the right therapy for his hyperactivity. Now, as a teacher, he is well-adjusted and helps children, many of whom have some of the same symptoms he dealt with when he was in school.

The labeling of psychiatric disorders itself is a subject of much controversy in the field of mental health and psychiatry, and both

1

professionals and individuals with mental health difficulties have objections and reservations.

David Rabiner, Ph.D. of Duke University, is an ADHD researcher at the forefront of evaluating scientific information and clinical studies on ADHD. Rabiner represents a moderate view of ADHD medication, presenting all sides of the issues involved, and has provided material for this book on the subject of medication for ADHD, as well as providing supplementary information on childhood depression, which is often comorbid or overlapping with symptoms of ADHD. Because depression is common with ADHD treatment, and pharmaceutically treated ADHD sometimes results in depression or in the prescribing of antidepressants, the subject of antidepressants, especially for children and teens, is given some consideration here.

Additionally, a synopsis of an Iowa State University study is included in the supplementary material section, which provides scientific support for the view that violent video games can affect a child's level of aggression, as well as contribute to symptoms of ADHD, something that has been observed by many, but that has been lacking in actual proof up until this point.

Joel Nigg, Ph.D., of Michigan State University, who graciously helped in the early stages of putting together the material that led to this book, and who authored the book, *What Causes ADHD?*, suggested in his book that playing violent video games might be a contributing factor to symptoms of ADHD and to the actual disorder. (Professor Nigg provides support for the idea that there are a wide range of factors, including environmental, that might contribute to ADHD, providing scientific evidence, as well as suggesting that a number of factors need to be further researched, including children's television habits in terms of content and quantity). Since the time of Dr. Nigg's research, there seems to be more direct evidence for the link between video game play and ADHD. Russell Barkley, Ph.D., whose work is referred to in this book, also kindly provided guidance and offered opinions which led to the formulation of some of the material here.

There are many others whose work has been used in connection with this book, and it is hoped that this information can help parents specifically, to help their children overcome symptoms of ADHD without medication, and that it might help some teachers and child study teams to take a more moderate approach towards medicating children.

Even if a parent chooses to have his child take medication for ADHD, the principles in this book can be of value, and can help the child to experience symptoms to a lesser degree. There is no book that provides all the answers to any medical, psychological or behavioral problem. However, educating oneself with various viewpoints and perspectives is the course of wisdom, and can contribute to a greater chance for success.

Chapter 1

What is ADHD?
Symptoms of ADHD
ADHD & School
The Controversy of Labeling
Single Parent Families
What Causes ADHD?
ADHD & Bipolar Disorder
Child Abuse
Sleep Disorders
Prevention, Prenatal Care

"We've gotten used to taking pills for much that ails us. But prescription drugs are not infallible and many have been pulled from the market or slapped with a warning by the FDA, due to health-threatening side effects. We don't lack for alternatives. Plenty of research shows that exercise, diet, and other lifestyle changes are effective weapons..."

"Let's be honest: there's a wonderful convenience to taking a pill. It's just so much easier than changing what we eat, mustering up the time and willpower to exercise..."

From: *Beyond pills: 5 conditions you can improve with lifestyle changes. Harvard Health Newsletter*

What is ADHD?

Jennifer's son Matt had always been difficult. He would tear through the house like a tornado, shouting, kicking and jumping off furniture. Nothing kept his interest for longer than a few minutes, and he would often run off without warning and mid-sentence, unconcerned about bumping into anyone or anything.

Jennifer was exhausted, but when Matt was in preschool, she wasn't too concerned because she guessed, "boys will be boys."

However, it was a struggle to try to get Matt to cooperate, and when he entered the third grade, his disruptive behavior and inattention in class raised the red flag of his teacher. Jennifer took Matt to the pediatrician, who, after a short interview, informed Jennifer that Matt most likely had ADHD. The best thing would be to prescribe stimulant medications, which he might not need to take for the rest of his life, but most likely for the rest of his school years at the least.

Jennifer was relieved and concerned at the same time. While she was happy to hear that Matt had a diagnosable condition, the prospect of her son being on medication for five or more years distressed her. Was medication really necessary? and, Is ADHD a real disorder?, were some of her questions. Also, what about the side effects? What would the medication do to his body? The pediatrician reassured Jennifer that everything would work out fine, and sent her home with a prescription.

Summary of Symptoms Associated with ADHD

These are some of the symptoms commonly associated with ADHD:

- *Poor concentration, distractibility, impulsive behavior, careless mistakes, difficulty in controlling anger, inability to complete tasks, difficulty sustaining attention towards tasks.*

- *Hyperactive behavior, excessive activity, fidgeting, squirming, running, climbing excessively.*

- *Poor listening skills.*

- *Talking excessively, blurting out answers before hearing the whole question.*

David Rabiner, of Duke University, an expert on ADHD, describes Attention Deficit Hyperactivity Disorder (ADHD), as *"a disorder characterized by a persistent pattern of inattention and/or hyperactivity/impulsivity that occurs in academic, occupational, or social settings."*

Some of the problems associated with ADHD include, making careless mistakes, failure to complete tasks, difficulty staying organized and becoming easily distracted.

Other issues are associated with hyperactivity, such as fidgetiness and squirminess, running excessively or climbing, inability to exercise self-control or sit still in class, inappropriate or excessive talking, being constantly on the go, impulsivity and impatience, difficulty waiting one's turn, blurting out answers in class and frequent interrupting, among other problems.

Rabiner explains that *"Although many individuals with ADHD display both inattentive and hyperactive/impulsive symptoms, some individuals show symptoms from one group but not the other."*

Who is affected by symptoms of ADHD?

- ADHD is usually considered to be a childhood condition, but ADHD symptoms can be present with adults as well.

- ADHD symptoms are manifest with poor concentration, impulse control, lack of attention or focus. ADHD sometimes includes hyperactivity, which may be the case in perhaps 40 to 70% of ADHD diagnoses.

- 3 to 10% of children in each state (U.S.) - 2.5 million school-age children, are diagnosed with ADHD.

- Up to 2/3 of children who are diagnosed with ADHD are also diagnosed with a wide range of secondary mental health disorders (comorbid) such as depression, an anxiety disorder, Tourette Syndrome, Oppositional Defiant Disorder (ODD) or Conduct Disorder (CD). (Ashley, S., 2005)

Since every child displays some of the symptoms associated with ADHD, when is ADHD diagnosed? Simply put, when symptoms are prolonged and disruptive to the daily life of the child (or adult) over an extended period of time.

ADHD and School

ADHD is most frequently initially addressed through the school system, although sometimes a parent or pediatrician might be the first to express concerns about apparent symptoms of ADHD. A teacher may often raise the first red flag. The child is evaluated and a child study team works with the child, teachers and parents, testing the child for ADHD. If a certain number of symptoms are considered to reach a level of intensity and duration to the point that it interferes with a child's ability to sustain day to day activities over an extended period of time, this can result in a diagnosis of Attention Deficit Hyperactivity Disorder or Attention Deficit Disorder, a label of ADHD for the child.

The benefit of the diagnosis is that it enables educators and the child study team to give extra time and attention to the individual child. A personal assistant also might be made available. Parents can take appropriate measure to educate themselves and make adjustments in their parenting, and this might help to offset the child's predisposition towards hyperactivity or distractibility. Educators can also work at providing positive educational solutions for these individual students. The extra attention given to a child in many forms, along with adjustments that parents might make, often can be key factors in a child's improvement.

When educators and psychologists make a diagnosis of disorders such as ADHD, there is usually a certain amount of subjectivity in the interpretation of the symptoms, that is, it depends on how an individual psychologist or team views and interprets these symptoms. Computer aided tests are generally also interpreted subjectively, rather than being purely scientific. EEG test (*electroencephalogram*, that is the recording of electrical activity of the brain through electrodes on the scalp), do seem to provide a certain amount of corroboration with the observational diagnosis of ADHD, and though not full-proof, is one of several methods or tests that are or can be used in making the diagnosis.

Parents and teachers should note that It is generally recognized that stimulant medications do not usually, or necessarily, significantly increase grade performance of themselves. (Eide & Eide, 2006; Dogget, M., 2004). Those studies which attribute increased grade performance to medication, usually do not delineate between the benefits of the medication, and that of any of a number of other interventions being administered at the same time, giving a misleading impression that the positive academic gains are attributable to medication, when in fact, they may be the result of therapy, special education, increased attention being given to the child, the teacher's responsiveness, or other changes.

Labeling of Psychiatric Disorders

To be noted: Not all agree with the labeling system as it relates to many psychiatric disorders. (Eide, B.,et al., 2006; Shannon, S., M.D., 2007). A tendency has developed based on what is known as the "medical model" of psychiatry, which is the most common platform in 21st century psychiatry (and the latter part of the 20th century), but not necessarily universally accepted even in the professional community, (Olfiman, S., 2007), of labeling and medicating. Additionally, there are other models of psychology which more fully explain the various dynamics involved in the development of mental health disorders and for mental health in general.[1]

The medical model involves identifying the symptoms an individual displays, matching these symptoms to a list of symptoms as denoted in the DSM-IV, (DSM-5, 2012), the psychiatric book of disorders, and determining the appropriate label for the disorder. What is deemed to be the appropriate medication, and/or other treatments for that disorder, is then prescribed. Therapy is sometimes used in conjunction with drug treatment, however, in commonly practiced modern psychiatry based on the "medical model," therapy, educational remediation, parental training, psycho-education, or self-help, is often given secondary consideration, and sometimes given very little, if any, consideration. In reality, self help and lifestyle changes need to be considered with any psychiatric diagnosis, and in giving attention to these, many, or even most of the symptoms of ADHD can often be addressed.

Studies have indicated that children who spend time outdoors, as one example, receive benefits of a positive reduction in symptoms of ADHD as a result. (Kuo, F.E., Ph.D., Taylor, A., Ph.D., 2004). It is also possible that children who watch less television (or who spend less time playing video games), might also benefit in terms of a reduction in the intensity of symptoms associated with ADHD over the immediate and long-term. (Cristakis, D., 2004)

Some parents who have cut out television and video games for their children during the school week, have seen dramatic improvement in the ability of their children to concentrate on their schoolwork and focus. Some have found that improvement in diet results in a reduction of symptoms.

The label "ADHD," as considered in this book, is a practice that can be controversial, and that in some countries (such as Britain), has been resisted by the professional community up until fairly recently. (Britain has not been as readily disposed to prescribe medication for ADHD as has the U.S.) Additionally, the practice of labeling a person, "my son *is* ADHD," "my daughter *is* bipolar," is something that is not encouraged by

---

[1] See: Bronfenbrenner's Ecological Systems Theory. Dede Paquette – John Ryan. *National-Louis University.*

7

many, including advocacy groups and government mental health agencies. One Seattle teen who had bipolar disorder said that it helped her by changing the way she expressed her experience. By saying "I have bipolar" rather than "I am bipolar," it helped her to see herself as a "whole person," that "the illness was something" she "could live with, not something that defined my existence." (Johnson, Linnea, Spring 2012. *NAMI Voice*). Therefore, this book tries to avoid labeling those who have symptoms of ADHD as *being* ADHD, or even necessarily *having* ADHD, as if there is nothing that can be done about it other than cope, but rather as having symptoms which are associated with ADHD.

An excellent and balanced resource on the issue of labeling in mental health, especially as it relates to children and teens, is the book, *Please Don't Label My Child,* by Scott Shannon, Ph.D., a child psychiatrist with years of experience in helping children, with their parents, with a wide variety of psychiatric issues.

The *American Psychiatric Association's Diagnostic and Statistical Manual-IV, Text Revision DSM-IV-TR*, is used by mental health professionals to diagnose mental health disorders. ADHD refers to attention deficit hyperactivity disorder, and what has been commonly referred to in the past as ADD, or attention deficit disorder. The DSM-IV-TR breaks down ADHD into three sub-classifications: **ADHD, Combined Type;** which includes symptoms typical of ADHD, along *with* hyperactivity and impulsivity; **ADHD, Predominantly Inattentive Type**, what has been referred to in the past as ADD, or attention deficit disorder, *without* significant hyperactivity or impulsivity; **ADHD, Predominantly Hyperactive-Impulsive Type**, when distractibility and inattentiveness is *not* significant. See: *Center for Disease Control and Prevention (CDC)*, Attention-Deficit / Hyperactivity Disorder (ADHD) - Symptoms and Diagnosis. The revised edition, DSM-V is available at the time of the publication of this book.
See: http://www.psych.org/mainmenu/research/dsmiv/dsmv.aspx

"...But the label—and the treatment—wouldn't have touched the true stress at the heart of Melanie's problem: her lack of connection with her overworked and emotionally unavailable parents. Please Don't Label My Child, Scott Shannon, M.D., p.20.

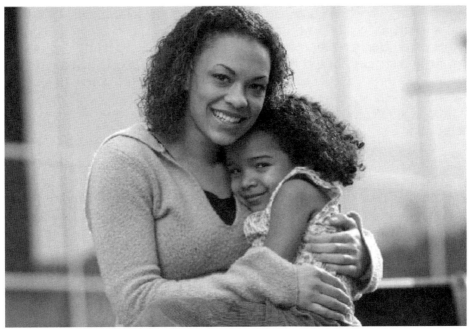

Single Parent Families

A disproportional number of children from single parent homes are diagnosed with ADHD. Poor family structure can be a factor. (Bee, H., et al., 2007). Lack of appropriate limits in the home can contribute to problems in school. However, other factors can be involved. Children need love, time and attention from parents, as well as strong emotional attachments. When these are lacking, it can contribute to behavioral and attentional problems in school and elsewhere.

Many sincere single parents struggle to make a living and to provide a loving home in which to raise a child. The challenges of both working and raising a family can leave one with little energy at the end of the day, and it can be challenging to meet both the physical and emotional demands of raising children. This can make it difficult for some parents to provide the ideal situation for their children. (Hill, K., 2006). Some single parents, then, may face difficulties balancing the emotional needs of their children, with the struggle to make a living, especially if they have several children. Grandparents and other caregivers may also face unique challenges in this regard.

Many principals and teachers are a source of unconditional love and support for children who might not otherwise receive love, tolerance or approval. Because teaching style can make a significant difference in the life and success of a child, teachers are encouraged to be patient and to help children to succeed, as well as avoid being unreasonable or harsh. Children are often in school for the better part of the day, many are in after-school programs, including programs which help children with homework.

Much is expected of teachers in terms of helping children to perform well academically, but it must also be noted that there are factors in school, at home, and in the community, which can contribute to a child's difficulties in succeeding academically and in the classroom. There are multi-faceted dynamics involved in a child's success, and this is most likely true with mental health issues, such as ADHD, and others, as well. (See Urie Bronfenbrenner's Bioecological Model of mental health, in contrast to the "medical model" of mental health, commonly used as a basis for labeling and drug treatment). (Paquette, D., Ryan, J., 2001. National Louis University). The classroom environment itself can affect the ability of some children to concentrate.

What Causes ADHD?

Joel Nigg, Ph.D., author of the scientifically-oriented book, *What Causes ADHD?*, who is an associate professor of psychology at Michigan State University, develops the idea that the causes for ADHD can be many and varied, but that there are causes. Some of these can be:

Prenatal

- Prenatal exposure to drugs, alcohol and smoking.
- Prenatal exposure to some prescription drugs.
- Babies born prematurely have a greater risk of symptoms associated with ADHD.

Genetic factors - Children may be born with a predisposition towards the symptoms of ADHD or depression. Other children in the same household, who are not genetically predisposed, might not develop these same symptoms.

Environmental factors - There is some evidence that certain environmental contaminants can contribute to the development of symptoms of ADHD in certain children. Some which are mentioned by name are PCBs, lead and mercury overexposure or poisoning. (Nigg, J., 2006).

Causes of ADHD, continued

Social factors

Social factors - Social isolation, or the need for friendships and positive (non-electronic) recreation, might also be contributing factors in some of the symptoms associated with ADHD for some children.

At home - The need for strong emotional attachments, or lack thereof, can contribute to symptoms of ADHD. Family problems, family instability, or a disorderly home can be contributing factors in some children's inability to concentrate or focus.

In the Classroom - There is some evidence that an improvement in classroom environment might help some children to better focus in class. Symptoms of ADHD which are strong in one classroom, might not be so pronounced in another. (Rabiner, D., March 2010; See also, *Focusing on Instruction, Teach ADHD*).

Physical Needs

Good diet and proper nutrition, regular meals each day, as well as exercise, can make a difference for children and teens with ADHD symptoms. Adults who are diagnosed with ADHD, or any mental health disorder, should give attention to these important areas of life. This can also be true for depression. Diets low in sugar and low in refined carbohydrates can have value for good general health, but can also contribute to good mental health.

This can mean doing without donuts, cakes, candy, cookies, white flour, white rice - instead, eat whole-grain foods, brown rice, whole wheat flour and healthy snacks, as a general rule of thumb, and without taking the area of diet to extremes. Children surprisingly love snacks like carrot and celery sticks, even in school. Don't confine your fruits to apples, bananas and oranges. Treat yourself and your children to the more exotic varieties of fruit. This can help hook them on eating healthy foods and can help some children with symptoms of ADHD. Eating healthy is a good practice for health and mental health regardless. Providing children with regular, healthful breakfasts, lunches, as well as snacks that are natural, rather than highly-processed foods, which may have many added chemicals and additives, can make a positive difference. Mayo Clinic states that while it is unlikely that food additives *cause* ADHD, it is possible that hyperactivity might be aggravated by some food additives. Other sources seem to agree.

Children and teens really do need to eat *three* healthful meals a day. While it might seem as if that goes without saying, a surprising number of children and teens don't eat regular meals. A healthy, regular breakfast is essential for a child's ability to concentrate in school. If a child skips breakfast regularly or regularly eats high-sugar foods, it can contribute to some of the symptoms of ADHD and/or depression for children who may have that genetic predisposition, especially when present with other contributing or aggravating factors.

Girls who are diagnosed with ADHD, are more likely to be of the inattentive type, boys tend to be hyperactive (Mayo Clinic). It stands to reason, that for a girl who does not eat regularly, doesn't eat breakfast and skips other meals, lack of proper nutrition might be contributing to her symptoms of inattention. This has been observed and noted in the classroom. School nurses, knowledgeable and authoritative on this subject, can and do talk with students who need help in this area.

In Newark, NJ, as one positive example, the implementation of a school breakfast program resulted in a 95.7% participation rate during the 2008-9 school year. School breakfasts went from 8,000 a day in 2004 to 25,000 per day during 2008-9. Other cities of note were Columbus, OH, and Boston, MA. (Essex News, February, 2010).

One of the problems, though, with school breakfasts, is that many are of very low nutritional value and high in sugar content: Fruit Loops, Apple Jacks, sugary muffins, Pop-Tarts, etc. There needs to be effort in many school districts to provide a consistently more-nutritious breakfast to children, one that is consistent with the health education that children and teens receive in class. Some school districts have made efforts along these lines, and some parents' groups have campaigned for better nutrition in their schools' menus.

Media - Long hours with the media, television, movies, video games, and Internet might affect the mind and behavior of many children. Content, such as violent content (Nigg, J., 2006), excessive action-violence or cartoon violence, as well as regularly watching horror movies, or pornography[2] and other sexually disorienting material, might also be factors which contribute to symptoms of ADHD, depression, or bipolar disorder, for some children, teens (or adults).

---

[2] Parents, stepparents, guardians, and anyone who works with children should realize that exposing under-age children to pornography or other non-educational sexual material may be considered a form of child abuse or gross neglect in some states. Many states have mandatory reporting laws for any form of suspected child abuse.

ADHD, bipolar disorder, and other disorders or conditions with similar symptoms

Symptoms that are evident with an ADHD diagnosis can also manifest themselves in disorders such as bipolar disorder. One clinical psychologist in a public school candidly acknowledged that *"it is difficult to accurately diagnose disorders [such as ADHD and bipolar disorder] in children because the symptoms of [several various] disorders overlap. The same symptoms often manifest themselves in different disorders."*

Mayo Clinic states that there are symptoms that resemble ADHD in the following disorders or conditions: learning or language problems, mood disorders (such as anxiety or depression), hyperthyroidism, seizure disorders, fetal alcohol syndrome, vision or hearing problems, Tourette Syndrome, sleep disorders and autism. Also of note, some of these disorders are diagnosed in as many as one in three children diagnosed with ADHD.

Psychiatrists might treat a client for both ADHD and bipolar disorder, or might mistakenly prescribe medications through an inaccurate diagnosis. Misdiagnosis is not uncommon. One of the reasons for this is that evaluations are most often subjective rather than being objective or scientific. In one recent study, it was concluded that over half of the clients being treated for bipolar disorder were misdiagnosed. (Zimmerman, M, M.D., 2007-9). The point of this being, that psychiatry is not an exact science, but there is much room for personal interpretation and error, by mental health professionals.

Zimmerman and his colleagues came to this conclusion through a more accurate, scientifically-oriented analysis of the symptoms of each respondent than is usually the case. What was apparently true, in this study, of bipolar disorder of over- or misdiagnosis, may also be true of ADHD as well, suggests Sharna Olfman's research in *No Child Left Different*. Olfman is a clinical psychologist and associate professor of psychology at Point Park University in Pennsylvania. David Rabiner highlights one clinical study indicating that there may be a 17% over-diagnosis of ADHD in children.

ADHD is not life threatening

ADHD poses no imminent danger to a child. A child might be more accident prone, but with a little extra attention by parents, this needn't be a major concern, and the probability of medicine fixing that problem is not certain. Of encouragement to parents is what is stated by author and ADHD authority Russell Barkley, that ADHD is not "a pathological condition or a disease stage". Rather, it is a "natural or developmental form" of the disorder ADHD, and then, *"should not be considered some grossly abnormal pathological condition."*

Instead, ADHD is described as a condition that is *"not qualitatively or categorically different from normal at all, but likely to be the extreme lower end of a normal trait. Thus the difference is really just a matter of degree and not a truly qualitative difference from normal."* Barkley states, *"this should help everyone view ADHD from a kinder perspective."* (Barkly, R., 1997).

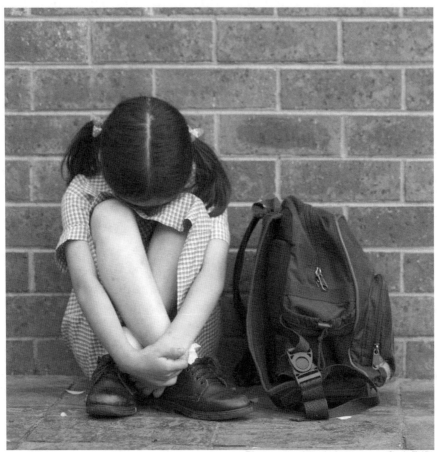

Photo: www.istockphoto.com   CraigRJD

Mistaken Identity: Child abuse and sleep disorders are often misdiagnosed as ADHD

Child Abuse – Children who have been sexually abused have mistakenly been treated for ADHD or bipolar disorder. Treatment and care for children who may have been victims of child abuse of any type is much different than the treatment for ADHD or bipolar disorder. Therefore, caregivers and professionals need to be very discerning before recommending pharmaceutical treatment.   Recovery from child abuse is

14

never as simple as prescribing a pill, and requires a multi-dimensional, long-term-effort. Support, therapy, and especially love and acceptance, are critical for recovery. A peaceful home life, stability, approval and reassurance are of necessity to the extent that is possible, from family, caregivers, teachers and mentors.

Children with sleep disorders have also been mistakenly treated with medications for ADHD. Children who are having trouble sleeping are often misdiagnosed with ADHD.

There can be many reasons that children are having difficulty sleeping and there can be practical solutions as well. One counselor recommends a "wind down" period, one hour before going to bed. Also, keeping the television, video games and Internet out of the bedroom can be of help to many children. Making sure children do not view stimulating movies or play stimulating video games before bedtime can be of help. (Walker, S., 1998).

Children need exercise, as do adults. Healthy outdoor activities are demonstrated to help many children with symptoms of ADHD and depression, as well as being an aid in helping a child or adult to sleep better at night. (Armstrong, T., 1997).

Children often outgrow symptoms of ADHD

Of encouragement for parents of children with ADHD symptoms, is that up to 35%, some say 50%, of children and teens who have the symptoms labeled as ADHD, outgrow these symptoms and no longer fall within a classifiable range, as a matter of course. (Barkley, R., 2008, p.49).

Symptoms and behavioral issues may be most difficult for the teacher in the classroom, or sometimes for the parent, but ADHD seldom poses imminent danger to the child or to classmates.

Prevention: Pregnant women who smoke, drink alcohol or abuse drugs put their future children at greater risk for ADHD. Adequate prenatal care, proper diet when pregnant, and regular visits to the doctor are essential. Breast feeding may also help the baby to bond with the mother and the mother to the baby, and this can be another effective preventive measure. [3]

---

[3] Rapley, G., October 5, 2002. Keeping mothers and babies together--breastfeeding and bonding. *RCM Midwives.* www.ncbi.nlm.nih.gov/pubmed/12851979

Child and Adolescent Mental Health and the Media

Video game play contributes to symptoms of ADHD.
Iowa State University researchers

Drawing helps kids to focus, in contrast to watching television cartoons. University of Virginia Researchers

Major Depression is associated with increased time listening to popular music, for adolescents. Researchers at the University of Pittsburgh

Major Depression in adolescents is reversely correlated with time spent reading print media such as books. University of Pittsburgh

Chapter 2

The Media and ADHD
Media: Television, Movies, Video Games, Music, Internet
Parental Training
Problems and Solutions

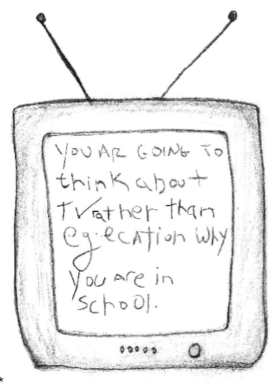

*

"We must be willing to look at any and all aspects of a child's life that seem to be off-kilter and not just focus on the symptoms that are most apparent to adults. In my practice, I find that I can do the most good if I don't apply a diagnostic label at all." Scott M. Shannon, M.D. Pediatric psychiatrist.

---

* Reproduction of young grade school child's work

Studies indicate that children who play video games on school days have lower grades than children who do not.[4]

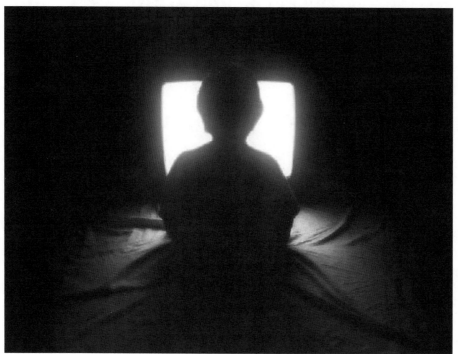

Photo: Aaron Escobar

Excessive time watching television and movies has been shown, in some clinical studies, to have a correlational relationship with symptoms of ADHD in children. Content might also be a factor.

[4] Cummings, H., 2007, as reported in the *Archives of Pediatrics and Adolescent Medicine. American Academy of Pediatrics.*

Television & Movies

The fast-paced imagery of television is believed to have a connection, with a reasonable degree of certainty, with attentional problems in children. This is especially true with regards to young children. One study concluded that for every hour a day that a child watched television, his or her chances of manifesting the symptoms of ADHD as an older child increased by 18%. (Christakis, D., et al, 2004).

The content of what children watch also may have a bearing on their ability to concentrate. A study conducted by Iman Sharif, M.D., from the Department of Pediatrics, Children's Hospital at Montefore/Albert Einstein College of Medicine in Bronx, NY, and James Sargent of the Department of Pediatrics, Children's Hospital, Dartmouth Medical School, Lebanon, NH, concluded that there is a strong correlation with lower school grades and media time. The team recommended that parents limit weekday television and video game time to one hour or less a day.

Exposure to adult material, including R-rated movies and videos also was correlated with lower grades. The team further recommended restricting access to cable movies, R-rated movies and videos. (Sharif, I., et al., 2006). Too much television is likely to negatively affect grades on math and reading scores. (Parents Magazine, November 2005).

Violent films and television, (as well as violent cartoons), are being viewed by children as young as kindergarten and pre-kindergarten ages. In one classroom, 50% of first-graders watched films of extreme violence. For some, it has been noted, this can result in disorientation and inability to concentrate. This observation has been observed in many inner-city classrooms.[5] It is possible that long hours with television and movies might also contribute to symptoms of depression in some young children. (Sigman, A., PhD., pp. 5, 187-189, 193).

Excessive time spent with electronic stimuli

Most children spend between 2 ½ to 6.5 hours a day on the media, that is television, movies, video games, Internet, iPods, etc. The question posed, "Are Our Children Too Wired?," in a *Time Magazine* article is a valid topic. Children or teens often multitask, when watching television, talking on the cell-phone, and when using the computer or iPod, texting, making emails, (two or more activities at the same time). (Wallis, C., March 19, 2006). Long hours with the media in any form can also contribute to symptoms of inattention, distractibility, and other symptoms associated with ADHD.

---

[5] New Jersey Teaching Notes, 2005-2010.

Video Games

Roberto was 12 years old, he had been on medication for ADHD for over a year. Still, none of his teachers could handle him, and his parents didn't know what to do with him. His grades were still failing, and he had tried several different medications.

However, a point that had never been addressed was that when Roberto came home from school, he didn't do homework or socialize, but usually played hours of the most-violent video games, unsupervised and alone. Is it possible that these many hours playing video games alone, might be affecting his ability to sit still in class, concentrate on schoolwork or to be able to integrate socially with other students? This illustrates the need to address root causes, rather than to emphasize treating symptoms, when considering childhood behavioral and mental health issues.

****

Boys especially can be susceptible to spending long hours daily on video games. Video games can be addictive for many children and teens. This might also contribute to symptoms associated with ADHD. (During a classroom discussions on anxiety, one educator and counselor commented that children "don't really need video games," as fifth-grade students spoke of having two or three different types of video game units each.)[6] Parents can provide alternative mentally, physically, healthful and enjoyable activities for children, without needing to provide an assortment of mentally-disorienting video games to children. There are many options for entertainment that children often enjoy more than video games once they get used to the idea.

A school psychologist who had pre-teenage children of her own and who also works regularly with children who have symptoms of ADHD, says that after reading about the adverse psychological and possible adverse physical effects that video games can have on children and teenagers, took video games out of her home. Her children are of college age today and successful.[7]

Of course, not all video games are detrimental to children. An Iowa State University study on the subject acknowledges that some video games can have a positive affect on children's social skills, are pro-active, and many are educational. The most common use of video games for children and teens, however, is video games with action and action violence, driving cars recklessly or shooting one thing or another. If not pointed in the right direction, boys easily acclimate to long hours playing these type of games. Most boys in the inner-cities are regularly playing

---

[6] New Jersey Teaching Notes, 2006.

[7] Ibid.

very violent video games. Girls, by contrast, in school, tend to gravitate towards gentler video games when they play on the computer.

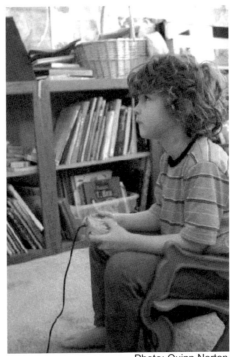

Photo: Quinn Norton

Time spent playing aggressive or violent video games might also have a correlation with symptoms of ADHD in some children.

Some pro-active games may be used in a school setting by educators, and educational games are available on the internet. However, parents need to choose video games for their children very carefully, directing their children towards games with a positive influence, preferably those of a slower pace, if they allow their children to play video games at all. This takes a great deal of effort on the part of the parent, and in some instances, it might be easier for parents to forgo video games for their children in the home, in lieu of other forms of recreation.

Many internet-based video games commonly played by children in public schools, advertised as "educational," are not in the least educational, but are labeled such because it is easier to get games which are labeled "educational" through the public school's internet filtering system (and other internet filtering software), and through the teacher's radar. (e.g. Does counting the number of bridges, tanks or apes you blow up with bombs or shoot, or the number of parachuting penguins you shoot down, really teach a 5th grader math?). At the best, such video games are mind-dulling, usually aggressive in one way or another, socially isolating and can sap up a child's limited time, a habit that follows many children through their adult years, even into marriage.

Movies and Children

Some children watch between one and three movies daily, every day, or as many as five or six movies in a single weekend. Fast-paced action movies and movies that feature the macabre or occult, scary, or horror movies, and otherwise violent movies, can be overwhelming to the minds of some children in their early childhood years. (Schmidt, B., M.D., 1991).

The artificial stimulation of movies and other intense forms of the media can overwhelm a child's senses and may also leave some children emotionally vulnerable, as well as making it difficult for some children to concentrate on regular school work, "sit still" in class or socially integrate pro-actively with other children. Noted child psychiatrist Peter Neubauer observed that the effects of movies which have disturbing content are usually more intense with children who come from poorly structured families. Lacking cohesion at home or positive emotional reference points, these disturbing scenes or themes in movies can result in further disorienting a child. (Neubauer, P., PhD).

Solutions

One educational psychologist in Paterson, NJ, concerned with what she described as "the epidemic" of ADHD cases in her school, encouraged parents to set firm limits for children in terms of television, video games and movies, as well as in other areas of life.[8]

Parental training programs have been recommended as a general positive intervention to help parents to fulfill their role as parents. Parental training can help parents, including single-parents, to care for, set limits, and in some cases, to learn how to raise and discipline children appropriately and effectively. (Hill, K., EdD. Paterson, NJ, 2005).

A 2012 clinical study with preschool children with ADHD, conducted by researchers from Queens College, NY has concluded that, *"consistently engaging children with ADHD in activities that challenge and exercise particular neurocognitive functions can strengthen the underlying neural activity that support these functions and thereby diminish ADHD symptoms." Journal of Attention Disorders,* March 15, 2012. *See p.76.*

---

[8] New Jersey Teaching Notes, 2006.

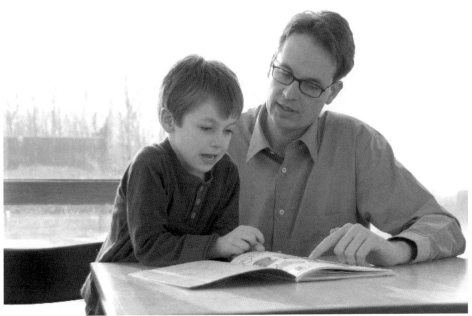

Children need firm limits and warm personal attachments

Parental Training

Parental training can help parents acquire new parenting skills and insight, which can result in a more-stable family structure for children. Small adjustments can make a big difference for some children who are struggling with symptoms associated with ADHD.

Newly acquired or refined parenting skills can result in the child's better coping with and even overcoming ADHD. The results may well result in lightening the load on the parents themselves, in the long run. Some community-based programs, religious organizations and public schools,[9] provide information, workshops, seminars or meetings for parents for this purpose. Utilizing such programs and training can benefit parents and children. Self-education through reading and study on the subject of parenting can also help.

Keisha Hill, Ed.S., a school psychologist, states with compassion, "Every day I talk to hard-working educators, parents, guardians, and grandparents who are calling out for help in dealing with children with ADD/ADHD. Regarding the classroom, teachers and staff would benefit from training in research-proven strategies for children with ADD/ADHD.

Furthermore, from what I have seen, these strategies are potentially beneficial to all students, even those without attention

---

[9] New Jersey Teaching Notes, 2010, Newark, NJ.

difficulties. However, the school cannot create optimal environments for ADD/ADHD in isolation. The home environment is very important. Although many parents are doing the best they possibly can to help their inattentive/hyperactive child and to just make it through the day without a tantrum or crisis, parent training groups have proven to be very effective.

For example, once parents understand that children with attention difficulties cannot self-regulate or 'keep everything together' as well as other children, they will need assistance [as] a parent with concepts such as decision-making, time-management and organization." Parental training is a valuable provision for many parents and children that can make a big difference in a child's long-term success.

Music

Teens are often deeply enamored with music and for some it can become an almost religious passion. (Crouse, J. S.. *Concerned Women for America)*. When this love for music is focused in a positive direction, it can provide wholesome recreation and contribute towards good mental health. For those who learn to play a musical instrument, for example, a child can gain a feeling of accomplishment and satisfaction, as well as self-esteem, as they make progress in developing their skills. (Timmes, A., 2005).

In some schools in Newark and Paterson, NJ, music teachers have educational programs whereby children can learn to play instruments such as the violin, something that children practice at home, and within six months time, most of the children in one noted public school program in Paterson, NJ, are playing very nicely. They are required to practice a half-hour a day at home, along with the time reserved for the activity a few times a week at school. Another middle school in Newark featured piano lessons for their students, with 10 or 15 electric pianos made available for classes and practice.

This can help children in their ability to focus and concentrate, as well as to develop a feeling of accomplishment and self-esteem. Similarly, while not necessarily scientifically proven at this point, children who are exposed to wholesome music from a young age might benefit in their cognitive ability and development.

On the other hand, the intense music that dominates much of the music scene today, especially if youths or children overdo it in terms of intensity or time spent on this form of entertainment, can sometimes contribute to problems with inattention, depression,[10] or contribute to the intensifying of some of the symptoms in some cases of bipolar disorder.

---

[10] Primack, MD, EdM, MS, et al., 2011. *Archives of Pediatric and Adolescent Medicine*.

There is, what would seem to be, an established connection between listening to intense music with strong emotional impact, as well as the amount of time spent doing so, with some mental health difficulties for some children, teens and adults. The music we listen to can affect the chemical balance of our brain, according to Joel Robertson, author of *Natural Prozac*. (Robertson J, PhD, 1998). This can be something positive if we are selective with our music.

The amount of time spent with music is something that parents and mental health professionals, as well as educators and principals, might need to give thought to. Some schools have incorporated strict policies in the school concerning iPod use and music during classes and in the halls. Moderation in music, then, can be part of the key for some teens. Exposing children and teens to music that is less intense, and to a wider variety of music which includes lighter music such as light classical or other mood and folk music, can have a beneficial and positive effect on children. Some teachers in the public schools do just that, and the strains and melodies of a wide variety of music can be heard from the classrooms of thoughtful music teachers who work hard to educate children in expanding their musical horizons,[11] as well as in the hallways of some high schools.

For children and youths who spend long hours with iPods, on the Internet with music, music videos and the radio, intensifying of symptoms associated with some childhood or teen mental health disorders might result. The mind is overwhelmed and cannot keep up with the intensity and fast pace that it is assimilating on a daily, even hourly basis. This, along with other factors, might contribute to symptoms of ADHD or depression in some children.

ADHD, then, may be the result of a genetic predisposition, along with any of a number of combinations of other factors, many of them which are controllable or adjustable.

---

[11] Rafael Hernandez Grade School and Malcolm X Shabazz High School, both in Newark, NJ, are two schools of note along these lines, although there are many others.

Learning to play a musical instrument such as,

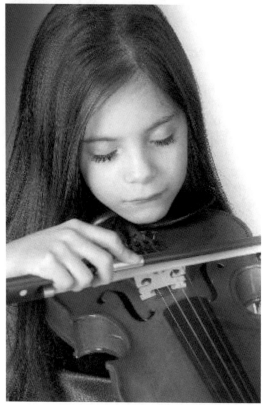

Photo: www.dreamstime.com Macromayer

*.......**violin or piano,** can help a child to develop self esteem* (Timmes, A., 2005), *as well as to develop his or her ability to concentrate.*

Chapter 3

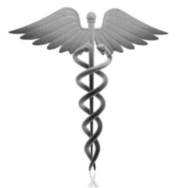

Is Medication the Answer?
Drug treatment, Amphetamines
Note from Center for Disease Control
and Prevention
Drugs have potential for abuse
Antidepressants
A realistic view of the benefits of
medication and side effects

It is generally acknowledged in the psychiatric and psychological professional communities that psychiatric medication treats symptoms, rather than the illness or the cause of the illness itself.

Psychiatric medication has been likened to an analgesic in that an analgesic does not address the cause of the pain, but merely assuages it.

Professor of psychology at Queens College, Jeffrey Halperin, who has researched ADHD for more than two decades states, "Much of the current data suggests that even kids who have been successfully treated with stimulant medications when they were young don't show lasting and long-term progress. Basically, drugs are only effective as long as they're being taken. Drugs don't have 'stickiness,' they don't persist". *(See p.76).*

******

The biggest reason parents are reluctant to prescribe medication for ADHD to their children is the side effects. Some of the side effects of ADHD medicine can include, "insomnia, anorexia, nausea, decreased appetite, weight loss, headache, increased blood pressure, faster pulse, abdominal pain and shifting moods. In some people, stimulants may cause involuntary muscle movements of the face or body (tics)." At times, not commonly, side effects can be more serious, including "seizures, high blood pressure (hypertension), delusions (psychosis) or liver problems." (Mayo Clinic, 2010).

******

"I'm not an enthusiast for attributing too much to an individual's biochemistry. I think that it is important for certain problems, but I think that the overselling of medication is one of the worse problems in the field, and it is getting worse all the time. Some psychiatrists now don't even seem able to talk to people - they only listen to decide which medications to prescribe. It's a shame." Noted Standford University therapist and founder of the Family Therapy Institute, Washington, D.C., Jay Haley. (Yatko, M., 2012).

In the decades of the 1960s and early 1970s until today, the medical model of psychiatry, and along with it the increasing use of psychiatric drugs for common mental health disorders, became the most common platform for psychiatric treatment. In the 1970s, stimulant drugs used for treating ADHD become widely used.

Drug treatment, along with counseling and therapy, have increasingly been employed as the front-line treatment for addressing ADHD (and depression) in the past few decades. Treating adults and children with medication for mental health difficulties and disorders has been and continues to be the subject of much controversy and conflicting clinical studies. (Kluger, J., 2003).

Stimulants are frequently prescribed for ADHD, and antidepressants have also become a secondary form of treatment when symptoms of depression become manifest in children. Symptoms of depression or clinical depression, after starting drug treatment for ADHD, does occur with some children. (Mental Health Weekly, 2004). It is possible that for some children, pharmaceutical treatment for ADHD might contribute to depression or to symptoms of bipolar disorder over time. (Olfman, S., 2007. p.58). Use of antidepressants might contribute to symptoms or diagnosis of bipolar disorder for some (children and adults).

Although drugs have been used for centuries in efforts to neutralize psychiatric disorders, including depression, widespread use of drugs for psychiatric disorders came into its own in the 1950s in psychiatric hospitals with the introduction of the drug commonly known as Thorazine, (chlorpromazine) which was administered as an antipsychotic to acute patients for schizophrenia and other psychotic disorders. It became the first widely-used typical antipsychotic. Typical antipsychotics that followed are much stronger in potency than Thorazine. (This is where the term "chemical straightjacket," or "chemical lobotomy" originated). Atypical antipsychotics with side effects less potent than typical antipsychotics, but strong nonetheless, were in the mainstream by the mid-1990s. Partly because the prescribing of such strong drugs, especially for vulnerable subsets of the population such as children, teens, foster children as well as adults and children on Medicaid, is often administered in an irresponsible manner, there is a strong counter-movement among professionals from the medical model towards a more balanced and responsible approach towards mental health treatment, including prevention, self-help and non-pharmaceutical professional therapies.

Drug Treatment for ADHD
Questions and Answers

Q - Do medications for ADHD have strong side effects?

A - Medications for ADHD, in general, do have strong side effects for most children. Approximately 90% of those who take medications for ADHD will experience strong side effects when they initially take the drug. However, the intensity of the side effects gradually lessens, so that within six months, only 50% will experience strong side effects, and by two years, only 15% will.[12]

Q - What are the side effects of stimulant medications?

A - There are side effects in the use of the vast majority of prescription drugs. With every benefit comes a risk. Parents, treating physicians and child study teams, must evaluate risks vs. possible benefits. Some of the less serious side effects for medications used in treating ADHD are, changes in weight and eating habits, (stimulants act as an appetite suppressant - some other psychotropic drugs have the opposite effect and lead to weight gain or even diabetes), difficulty sleeping, changes in mood.

Other side effects that have been mentioned are, robotic effects, lack of flexibility, workaholic tendencies, insomnia, a feeling that you are going to "jump out of your skin". Facial tic-disorders and the exacerbation of previously occurring tic-disorders can be side effects for a subset of children treated with stimulant medication. (6.4% of children with no previous history of tics reported new onset of tics with stimulant treatment, according to one study, and 2% discontinued stimulant treatment because of onset of new facial tics).[13] On the other hand, some have argued that tic disorders have developed with children with ADHD treated with placebos. There have been isolated instances of the actual development of Tourette Syndrome in association with the use of stimulant medications. (more details on facial tics on page 38).

Very serious side effects are experienced by less than one-percent of those who take the drugs, and include, schizophrenic-like symptoms, suicidality, or sudden death due to heart failure for those

---

[12] Rabiner, D., January 2006. *Attention Research Update* newsletter. Based on the following study: (Monastra, V.J. 2005. Overcoming the barriers to effective treatment for attention-deficit/hyperactivity disorder: A neuro-educational approach. *International Journal of Psychophysiology*, 58, 71-80).

[13] Palumbo D, Spencer T, Group CS: Impact of ADHD treatment with once-daily OROS® methylphenidate on tics. Program and abstracts of the Annual Meeting of the American Psychiatric Association; Philadelphia, Pennsylvania; 2002. As referenced in *Medscape Today News.* http://www.medscape.com/viewarticle/458811_2

(children) with undetected congenital heart defects. (Mayo Clinic, Aug. 2011). Side effects are the primary reason many parents are reluctant to prescribe medication for their children.

A clinical study released in 2009 and published in the American Journal of Psychiatry, examining the issue of sudden unexplained death for children and adolescents taking stimulants for ADHD, concluded that the odds of sudden unexplained death are six to seven times greater than the general population. The study concluded, *"Such an association is biologically plausible given the central and peripheral catecholaminergic effects of stimulants and significant increase in heart rate and blood pressure that accompany their use."* [14]

Q - Are there any who don't respond to ADHD medications?

A – Up to 42% of those who take medications for ADHD have no positive response, and for some, stimulant medication results in increased behavior problems.[15] It seems to be a similar rate for antidepressants, where approximately 60% do not respond to the first antidepressant prescribed (Science Daily, December 15, 2011), and up to 50% do not experience any improvement in depression with antidepressant use. (Virginia Commonwealth University Research, November 2011).

Q - Are the positive effects of medications for ADHD long-term?

A - For those who experience positive effects from drugs for ADHD, those effects have a parallel profile to the side-effect curve. They are generally effective over the short term, but their effectiveness in individuals gradually lessens over one to two years. (Rabiner, D., January 2006, *Attention Research Update*).

Q - Do clinical studies support the use of non-pharmaceutical methods in treatment of ADHD?

A - Yes, there are some clinical studies which indicate that "green therapy," as an example, time spent outdoors in a natural setting, playing in the park, etc., does have a positive affect on symptoms associated with ADHD, [16] and can also have positive effects for depression and for

---

[14] Sudden Death and Use of Stimulant Medications in Youths, (September 2009). Madelyn S. Gould, et al. *American Journal of Psychiatry*. 2009:166:992-1001. 10.1176/appi.ajp.2009.09040472

[15] Doggett, Mark, A., Ph.D., 2004. School of Education, Colorado State University. *Journal of Child Health Care*.

[16] "From our previous research, we knew there might be a link between spending time in nature and reduced ADHD symptoms, The greenest space was best at improving attention after exposure. if we kept everything else the same, we just changed the environment, we still saw a measurable difference in children's symptoms. And that's completely new. No one has done a study looking at a child in different environments, in a controlled comparison where everything else is the same." Andrea Faber Taylor, PhD, and Frances E. Kuo, PhD, University of Illinois. August, 2008 *Journal of Attention Disorders*.

anxiety. Clinical studies do indicate that exercise can be a very effective natural therapy for depression (Mayo Clinic, October 2011; Duke Today, Duke University, September 22, 2000), and that talk therapy for teens and some children does have benefit, and can also be a protective measure for some. Cognitive therapy for depression and ADHD can also be effective in many cases, as can ADHD coaching.

Cognitive behavioral therapy for depression has been demonstrated to have a positive benefit at the same general rate as medication[17] in the short-term, and is generally a better long-term solution. It can also be an effective therapy for ADHD. However, because pharmaceutical companies finance most of the studies being performed on the subject of treatment for mental health disorders, even those conducted by universities, there is a shortage of studies that have been conducted on non-pharmaceutical methods in the mental health field and in psychiatry in general. Studies which contradict the results the sponsoring company desires, are often left unpublished. [18]

Q - Do clinical studies support the view that medications for ADHD improve grades for children in school?

A - Results are mixed, but it has been concluded by some that grade performance is not significantly positively affected by medications for ADHD. Mark A. Doggett, Ph.D. of the School of Education, Colorado State University, states that a "meta-analysis of 74 studies" indicates that use of stimulant medication, "had little impact on educational outcomes." (Dogget, M.A., PhD, 2004). Parents, though, who are diligent in shielding

---

"After demonstrating that 30 minutes of brisk exercise three times a week is just as effective as drug therapy in relieving the symptoms of major depression in the short term, medical center researchers have now shown that continued exercise greatly reduces the chances of the depression returning." Septmeber, 2000. Michael Babyak, Steve Herman, Parinda Khatri, Dr. Murali Doraiswamy, Kathleen Moore, Teri Baldewicz, Duke University, Edward Craighead, University of Colorado.

---

[17] "Studies have shown that cognitive therapy is an effective therapy for depression and is comparable in effectiveness to antidepressants...Cognitive therapy has also proved beneficial in treating patients who only have a partial response to adequate antidepressant therapy...Good evidence has shown that cognitive therapy reduces relapse rates in patients with depression, and some evidence has shown that cognitive therapy is effective for adolescents with depression." Rupke, Stewart J., et al. Michigan State University College of Human Medicine, East Lansing, Michigan. *American Family Physician,* January 1, 2006.

[18] Less than 50% of studies funded or partially funded by the National Institutes of Health were published within 30 months, according to the Yale School of Medicine Researchers. *Science Daily,* January 3, 2012.

children from negative media influences such as violence in the media, may expect positive gains in grade performance. (Cummings, H., 2007).

Q - Does use of medications for ADHD lead to an increased risk of drug abuse?

A - While some medication studies may indicate that use of stimulant medications does not contribute to increased risk of drug abuse, it is possible that under certain conditions there may be an increased risk of drug abuse, although more research is needed.

On the one hand, methylphenidate (Ritalin) and stimulants themselves are highly abused drugs. In some studies, there may be indication that for the majority who use the drugs, it does not progress to abuse of illegal drugs at a disproportional rate. (Wiles, T.E., et al., 2003). On the other hand, a study reported in the *National Institute on Drug Abuse* reported that in animal studies, laboratory animals which had been exposed to methylphenidate as juveniles, develop a seven-times as great a rate of cocaine dependence, as those which had not, as adults. The results of this study were not replicated for infant laboratory animals exposed to methylphenidate, which seemed to have close to the same rate of cocaine dependence. (Williams, J., Zickler, P., June, 2003). The implication being, that there may be some physical or psychological connection between *adolescent* exposure to some stimulant drugs and future drug use potential. Again, more research is needed to isolate at-risk sub-groups for possible increased abuse of prescription stimulant drugs.

Amphetamines - Adderall (Dextro/levo-amphetamine) and Dexedrine (Dextroamphetamine) are amphetamines, widely prescribed for children in treatment for ADHD symptoms. Methylphenidate, most commonly prescribed as Ritalin, or in a long-lasting formula, Concerta, is the most well known medication for treating ADHD. Another medication that has been used is Cylert (pemoline) which is a long-lasting medication but that does not have the immediate affect of the amphetamines or of methylphenidate (Ritalin). (Reported cases of liver damage has caused the FDA to issue warnings with the goal to phase Cylert out of use in the U.S.; FDA Alert: Liver Injury Risk and Market Withdrawal, October, 2005).

"It's our job to listen to them attentively and openly, to resist labeling them, and to work to remove the stressors from their lives that are blocking their mental and emotional health." Scott M. Shannon, M.D.

"There are several public health concerns relative to pharmacotherapy. Pharmacologic treatment is extremely prevalent. Assessing the health risks and benefits to young children, particularly preschoolers, is a high priority. Children who begin medication therapies very early and receive treatment on a long-term basis may have unknown risks associated with current treatments. Additionally, pharmacologic intervention often do not normalize behavior. Research, albeit limited, suggests that even with long-term treatment, children and adults with ADHD experience substantial problems in the school, home, workplace, and community settings. This raises questions about the effectiveness of pharmacologic interventions as a long-term approach." Center for Disease Control and Prevention Department of Health and Human Services. U.S. Government agency. (www.cdc.gov)

"Behavioral Modification" is an approach that is recommended by the *Center for Disease Control and Prevention* for ADHD in children.

Stimulants work by raising the dopamine level of the brain. Cocaine has a similar chemical structure to stimulant medications. (Hallowell, E., Ratey, J., 1994), the main difference being that cocaine is released rapidly, creating a rush, whereas stimulants are released gradually over a long and controlled period of time. Therefore, the dopamine level is raised with stimulants, but not in the same rapid and addictive way as with cocaine. (Medicating Kids: Interview with Russell Barkley. *PBS, Frontline*).

Drugs have potential for abuse and caution must be exercised by parents, educators and physicians. One can become psychologically or physically dependent on prescription medications. Methylphenidate and other stimulants are among the most widely abused drugs. Withdrawal symptoms of prescription medications can be severe. Both physicians and those taking amphetamines, as well as parents whose children may be taking amphetamines, need to be very cautious in administering such drugs, as well as in protecting anyone in the household from abusing such prescribed drugs.

Methylphenidate is reportedly the fourth most widely abused drug, after marijuana, cocaine and heroin. It is not necessarily the individual to whom the drug is prescribed who is abusing it, although it can be, but the drug finds its way into the streets and is sold as a street drug or performance enhancer to college students and others.

"I have come to appreciate that medication ultimately treats symptoms, not problems," regarding psychiatric treatment. Psychiatrist Thad F. Ryals, M.D.

While it is commonly stated that 70% of those who take stimulant medications show improvement with drug treatment, it has been suggested that it is possible that much of the positive affect of drug treatment might be attributable to the therapy, support and attention that some children receive, in addition to the drug therapy, rather than being solely a result of the affect of the drug. Placebo response for ADHD is described, in a clinical trial conducted by Dr. Jeffrey Newcomb with the Mount Sinai School of Medicine, as being associated with a "robust" response, resulting in a 40% decrease in symptoms based on change on the total score of the ADHD Rating Scale for certain subgroups of ADHD.[19] The overall picture from other studies on the subject indicates that a positive response rate to placebos administered for ADHD positively affects 30% of children with ADHD. (Waschbusch, D.A., MD, et al., 2009).

The mere act of going to a doctor or even the attention from a caring nurse, a child's having someone that he or she can talk to about his or her situation, or that parents might be giving him or her more attention, is of benefit for many children, and reduces severity of symptoms associated with ADHD.

Additionally, there are few long-term studies concerning the effects of psychiatric medications on children and teens, including stimulant medications for ADHD. One comprehensive long-term study of ADHD treatment indicates that positive benefits of medication are negligible for most children within two years. (Rabiner, D., January, 2006. *Attention Research Update*). In other words, after taking the drugs for two years, stimulant medications no longer seem to make much of a difference for most children, although children can become dependent on them for normal functioning.

"Evidence suggests that parents and teachers tend to evaluate children with ADHD more positively when they believe the child has been administered stimulant medication and they tend to attribute positive changes to medication even when medication has not actually been administered." Daniel A. Waschbusch, PhD, William E. Pelham, Jr., PhD, James Waxmonsky, MD, Charlotte Johnston, PhD., (2009). Journal of Developmental & Behavioral Pediatrics.

---

[19] Newcomb, J., M.D., et al., August, 2009. Characteristics of Placebo Responders in Pediatric Clinical Trails of Attention-Deficit/Hyperactivity Disorder. *Journal of the American Academy of Child and Adolescent Psychiatry.*

Antidepressants

Antidepressants have been prescribed for over fifty years to treat depression. Tricyclic antidepressants, MAOIs, and more recently, SSRIs such as fluoxetine (Prozac) and many others, are used by millions, both adults, teens and children. Presently, only Prozac has been approved for use for children. However, often, until a contrary ruling by the FDA for a particular drug, doctors will prescribe certain psychiatric medications "off-label" to children, that is, outside of the FDA recommendation for the type of disorder the drug was intended, approved or tested for.

Antidepressants have been used by many for help in overcoming symptoms of depression and for slightly less than 50% of those who use them, they have been at least of some help. "*More than half the people who take antidepressants never get relief from their symptoms,"* concludes *Northwestern University Feinberg School of Medicine* in an article entitled Antidepressant Drugs Aim at Wrong Target. The article highlights new research on antidepressants.

The reasons for depression can be many and varied, therefore, it is to be expected that there would be different outcomes for different people.

The duration of the effectiveness of antidepressants varies from person to person. The expression, "Prozac Poopout," has been dubbed for the observation that there is a tendency for antidepressants to gradually or suddenly loose their effectiveness. (Lambert, C., 2000. The Downsides of Prozac. *Harvard Magazine*). This can happen within three to six months, or within a two to nine year period. For some, this can come in the form of a sudden crash, which can be intense and distressing. *Harvard Medical School in Harvard Health Publications* (2005), states that one of the risks of antidepressants is "**Loss of effectiveness.** Any antidepressant may lose its affect after months or years, sometimes because the brain has become less responsive to the drug."

Therefore, some psychiatrists and medical doctors have taken the viewpoint of using antidepressants only as a last resort in cases where there is a serious crisis in terms of danger to the client. The drug is used only as a temporary stop-gap until other issues such as lifestyle or trauma, that might be contributing to the depression, can be addressed, and never for more than a few months or as a lifestyle drug. (Glenmullen, J., M.D., 2000; Shannon, S. M.D., 2007).

One study from the Netherlands states that there is a *"significant association between degree of serotonin reuptake inhibition by antidepressants and risk of hospital admission for abnormal bleeding as the primary diagnosis.* "[20] The reason for this, the medical team states, *"Serotonin plays a role in platelet aggregation. Because antidepressants influence blood serotonin levels..."* Additionally, some specific types of antidepressants quadruple the risk of receiving a blood transfusion (because of abnormal bleeding).[21] All of the long-term physical effects of antidepressants have not yet been determined.

The growing use of antidepressants and stimulants for young children, as early as preschool and kindergarten, is something of growing concern. If statistics are accurate, approximately nine-percent of all children in the United States are taking psychiatric medications (six million children taking psychiatric medicine, out of a total of approximately 63 million children and teens, 3 to 17 years old, in the U.S.). (The Medicated Child. January 8, 2008. *Frontline, PBS;* ChildStates.gov).

A significant percentage of youths (adults and children) have been on, and are being prescribed, what are described as prescription "cocktails," that is, four, five or more different prescriptions prescribed at one time to achieve results, or to address various perceived psychiatric diagnoses or labels.[22] This is not, of course, the case in treating ADHD, but it is a related topic, in that new symptoms often develop, once one buys into the medical model, and can lead to the prescribing of stronger and stronger drugs, as new diagnoses are reached. In other words, what starts out as a simple prescription for a stimulant, can end up, in time, becoming a series of prescriptions for multiple drugs other than stimulants for other disorders which develop.

Strong side effects, such as extreme drowsiness and lethargy, are compounded with use of multiple medications. Some studies have concluded that there is no apparent benefit in the adding of more than one drug to a child or adult's drug regimen. (Sachs, G., 2007).

George Albee, Ph.D., professor emeritus of the University of Vermont, was a prominent psychologist and former president of the American Psychological Association (APA), and up until his death, wrote extensively on the subject of prevention in mental health, and of the value of addressing social stressors in the diagnosis and treatment of mental health disorders. Albee felt that this was especially true with regards to

---

[20] Welmoed E. E. Meijer, PhD, et al., (November 22, 2004). *Archives of Internal Medicine.* 2004;164:2367-2370.

[21] Movig, Kris L., et al., (October 27, 2003). Relationship of Serotonergic Antidepressants and Need for Blood Transfusion in Orthopedic Surgical Patients. *Archives of internal Medicine.* 2003;163:2354-2358.

[22] Sparks, J., University of Rhode Island; Duncan, B., The Ethics and Science of Medicating Children. Ethical Human Psychology and Psychiatry, Volume 6, Number 1, Spring 2004.

children. His view seemed to be that pharmaceuticals in the treatment of mental illness should not be used in treating children, and should not be emphasized with adults. (Remembering George Albee., 2006. *Society for Community Research and Action*).

For those who wish to stop using antidepressants, or any psychotropic drug, many sources indicate that they should do so gradually, rather than abruptly. (Kelly, R., 2005). Dr. Joseph Glenmullen is a psychiatrist who has written two books on the subject, *Prozac Backlash* and *The Antidepressant Solution*. Glenmullen describes his books as guides that can be used along with your doctor in an effort to successfully reduce an antidepressant prescription, with the goal of eventually doing without it.

Summary of serious side effects for stimulant medications

Serious side effects are possible with use of stimulant medications. The risk of serious side effects increases with the use of multiple medications. The percentage of children and youth who have serious side effects to stimulant medication decreases in time. Up to 90% will initially demonstrate what is considered to be serious side effects with use of medications commonly used in the treatment of ADHD symptoms. In six months time, the rate declines to about 50% and within two years on stimulant medications, the rate further decreases to around 15%. *(The rate of effectiveness for stimulant medications also seems to decline over the same period of time, almost proportionately to the side effect rate).* [23]

About 40% will show no response to medication, and around five to ten-percent are intolerant to any form of pharmaceutical treatment for ADHD. In the case of very serious side effects, such as schizophrenic-like symptoms, risk of suicide or sudden death due to heart failure, which has been reported with some stimulant medications, the rate is less than one-percent.

"Very often medication treats symptoms only..." regarding the use of psychiatric medications in the treatment of various types of psychiatric disorders. *Handbook of Clinical Neurology,* 1985. Quote from Jean Constantinidis and Jacques Richard, University Department of Psychiatry, Medical School of Geneva.

---

[23] Interpolated from *Attention Research Update*, David Rabiner, PhD., 2006.

Tic Disorders, Increased Aggression
and Stimulant Medicines

Some studies indicate that stimulant medication may result in an increased risk of tic-disorders, that is, facial tics, in up to nine-percent of those who take stimulant medication.[24] Additionally, pre-existing tic-disorders might be exacerbated by the use of stimulant medications. Tourette Syndrome has developed in a small number of children or youths who have begun stimulant medication treatment. In most cases, tic-disorders abate when treatment is suspended.[25] While tic disorders are a real concern for parents, also to be considered is that some studies have concluded that the rate of tic-disorders as a result of stimulants is not significantly higher in children with ADHD, than that with placebo treatment.

A recent study (2008) concluded that methylphenidate may increase hostility and possibly aggression, in children who take the drug for ADHD. (King, S., et al., 2008).

Additionally, forcing or coercing a child to take psychiatric medication is something that is not recommended by a number of mental health professionals. (Mate, G., MD, 1999). This can cause some children to become rebellious, resentful, or to distance themselves emotionally from a parent. The effect on the child of forcing the child who is unwilling, to take medication, is considered to be worse than that of the symptoms associated with ADHD in such cases. Two noted psychiatrists, John Ratey, M.D. and Edward Hallowell, M.D., experts in the field of ADHD, commenting in their book on the subject of ADHD, explain that children should not be forced to take medication, but should take the drugs of their own volition, as forcing a child to take drugs for ADHD could be damaging to the child psychologically in the long term. (Hallowell, E., Ratey, J., 1994).

Commenting on the effectiveness of psychoeducation in mental health treatment, Fahriye Oflaz Ph.D., Sevgi Hatipolu, Ph.D. and Hamdullah Aydi, M.D., state in a paper published in the *Journal of Clinical Nursing*, that psychiatric *"medication treats symptoms."*[26]

---

[24] Wilens, T., et al., 2006. *Archives of Pediatric and Adolescent Medicine.*
[25] Mick, E. The relationship between stimulants and tic-disorders in children treated for attention deficit hyperactivity disorder. *Harvard School of Public Health.*
[26] The specific disorders that the paper was addressing were depression and post traumatic stress disorder, (PTSD) but the principle also applies to ADHD.

Chapter 4

Other Solutions to ADHD
Green therapy
Exercise
Art
Professional Art Therapy
Love

Questions to ask

- *What, If anything, seems to worsen symptoms?*
- *What, if anything, seems to help in diminishing symptoms?*

"As an art educator with AD/HD, I have been both a student with AD/HD, and a teacher of students with AD/HD. In the public schools [and at the college level], the art room is often the one place where others with AD/HD feel at home. The point is that when kids with AD/HD find [or create] an environment supportive of their needs, the AD/HD becomes a non-issue, and in some cases, an asset. By harnessing their creative energy and finding a productive outlet for their intelligence, the possibilities are endless. The potential for success and the enjoyment of life is enormous! To those with AD/HD, I recommend flipping the coin and embracing what you find on the other side." Daniella Barroqueiro, Ph.D., Illinois State University, 2006.

Are There Other Treatment Solutions to Symptoms of ADHD?

Yes. Some have found success with their children in reducing the amount of time spent watching television, movies and video games to the greatest extent possible. The conclusion of one special education teacher who commented succinctly on her view of children's behavioral and attentional difficulties in school, was that most students had difficulty concentrating because of "the media".[27] The average time spent on the media for children and teens is between 2 1/2 to 6 1/2 hours a day. (Wallis, C., 2006). (In the school in which this special education teacher worked, one student reported that her sister played video games up to 16 hours in one day). That rate actually has increased, according to the most recent reports, by as much as 15% since this statistic of 2 1/2 to 6 1/2 hours was reported in 2005.

- One father with a large family kept video games put away in the closet during school months.[28] His children were diligent in doing their homework, even when the father wasn't home to supervise them.

- One parent limited television time to one-half hour a day for her young children, while providing other forms of wholesome recreation for the children, along with encouragement for the children to spend more time reading. Another parent does not allow cable television in his home (he lives in a region where only cable TV is available) because of the violence that is common in programming for children.[29]

  Taking the television and video games (as well as open access to the Internet) out of the bedroom of a child or teen can also be of value for many who have attentional difficulties.

- A father whose nine-year-old son was struggling with attentional problems and whose grades were suffering as a result, restricted television and video games to the weekends during school months for both his children. While the children were reportedly a little antsy the first two weeks, soon, the time they had spent with TV and video games became filled with outdoor

---

[27] New Jersey Teaching Notes, 2008.
[28] South River, NJ, 2006.
[29] Pennsylvania, U.S.

activities, playing together and reading. The improvement in schoolwork as well as the ability to read and concentrate for the attention-deficit nine-year-old was nothing short of remarkable. The boy achieved the honor role within six months. He had received a few months of tutoring during that period and prior. Previously, he had difficulty concentrating on and performing the simplest math problems for his age group and was at least a year behind in his math level.[30] This circumvented the need to experiment with stimulant medications.

What About Diet?

One reading coach who works with learning disabled children, including children who display the symptoms of ADHD, says that the first thing she encourages parents to do is to take their children off of a diet high in refined sugar.[31] It is possible that a poor diet might contribute to the intensity of some symptoms for some children with ADHD, or it may be a contributing factor for some of the symptoms, according to a spokesperson for CHADD.[32]

Some have concluded that it seems to be unlikely that a high sugar diet or diet alone causes ADHD for most children, but rather, it seems more likely that diet may be one of a number of contributing or aggravating factors. In one study, a meta-analysis of the effects of sugar on children's behavior and cognition concluded that, while such did not cause significant behavioral problems, "a small effect of sugar on subsets of children cannot be ruled out." (Wolraich, M. L., MD, et.al., 1995).

On the other hand, taking it from a positive viewpoint, rather than a causal perspective, changing diet can affect a positive response in children.

A 2009 study conducted by the ADHD Research Center in the Netherlands concluded that a "restricted elimination diet" reduced symptoms of ADHD in children with ADHD by 73%, compared to 0% for a control group. The study used parent and teacher ratings based on the abbreviated ten-item Conners Scale and the ADHD-DSM-IV Rating Scale. Interestingly, children with "comorbid symptoms of oppositional defiant disorder also showed a significantly greater decrease in ADHD symptoms" of 45.3%. The study concluded, "A strictly supervised elimination diet may be a valuable instrument in testing young children with ADHD on whether dietary factors may contribute to the manifestation of the disorder and may have a beneficial effect on the children's behaviour. (Pelsser L. M., Frankena, K., Toorman, J., Savelkoul, H. F., Pereir, A., Bultelaar, J.K. January 2009. A randomised controlled trial into the effects of food on ADHD. *European Journal of Child and Adolescent Psychiatry*).

---

[30] New Jersey Teaching Notes, 2008.
[31] McNuff, J., 2005. Paterson, NJ.
[32] Phone Interview, 2005.

Adjusting to a more-nutritious diet, then, for a child, can be a good and simple first or second step that parents can take. In fact, studies indicate that rather than following specific fad diets, adhering to a healthy diet has positive effects on mental health in general. Therefore, positive changes in diet and nutrition is part of a balanced plan for any mental health disorder or issue.

Obesity and problems associated with obesity among children due to poor dietary habits and lack of exercise is also of concern to many professionals and parents in recent years. (In India approximately 10% of all children are reportedly obese, with a correspondingly higher rate of diabetes).

Food additives may affect the mood or behavior of some children. Parents, though, should realize that there is rarely one factor that is causing symptoms associated with ADHD, but it is usually a combination of factors. Diet can be one of these factors. Focusing on something narrow such as food additives as the *cause* of ADHD might prove to be frustrating rather than constructive. So when it comes to diet, parents need to be balanced. Some food additives which are mentioned with reference to ADHD are benzoate, FD&C Yellow No.6 (sunset yellow), FD&C Yellow No.1 (quinoline yellow), FD&C Yellow No.5 (tartartrazine), FD&C Red No. 40 (allura red). (Huxsahl, J.E., M.D., 2010. Mayo Clinic).

If food additives are a real concern to some parents, they might consider purchasing only organic foods, which many do for a number of reasons. Organic foods have no additives, and purchasing them is a simpler measure than scrutinizing individual packaged foods purchased in a supermarket for specific additives, or testing a variety of specific additives for possible reactions. Organic food can typically add approximately 35% to 50%, or even more, to the grocery bill.

Children need breakfast, and for children who skip breakfast, their ability to concentrate in the classroom can be affected. Sugary cereals, which are frequently served as breakfast in school, can work in the opposite direction for some children, especially those whose metabolism might be sensitive, and cause them to lose the ability to concentrate well, as there is little nourishment in most sugary cereals. A healthy breakfast is a must for both young children and teenagers whose bodies are rapidly developing.

A low-sugar diet by avoiding sugars found in sugary cereals, soda, chocolate, and flavored milk,[33] candy, ice cream, cakes, sugary juices, etc., can have beneficial effects on general health, weight loss and mental health. An active rather than sedentary lifestyle can also help a child overcome many symptoms associated with ADHD. Schools may want to

---

[33] Chocolate and strawberry milk are served to children in public schools daily for lunch and are loaded with added sugar.

42

consider upgrading the quality of the food provided for children, which some public schools are giving attention to, by replacing sugary breakfasts and snacks with more-nutritious foods and foods which have a lower sugar content. This could prove to be beneficial in terms of the diabetes rate among children, better general mental health in children and teens, as well as in teaching children through example how to eat healthfully. Some children may be able to concentrate better in class more consistently.

In an effort to remedy this situation, some schools and parents' groups have worked together in formulating a program for more-nutritious meals for children in school (Moody, S., 2007), something which can significantly contribute to better classroom performance and behavior. Natural snacks such as fruit, wholewheat crackers with little added sugar, raw vegetables, fruit and other natural foods are a healthy alternative to high-sugar snack foods. When healthy snacks such as these are served in school, children take to it like a duck to water, rather than otherwise. For parents, serving healthy snacks to their children takes planning and forethought. This will help children and teens to concentrate better in class, can positively affect the behavior of some, and the blood-sugar level through a more healthful diet will be more stable in individual children. Their chances of developing diabetes as children or teens will be diminished. [34]

Also, these efforts in schools will help children to establish good life patterns, not just by what they read in textbooks, but by a positive example that is set in school for good nutrition.

A note on childhood and teen depression

The reasons for childhood depression, or any form of depression, like ADHD, are many and varied, and every child and teen is different. Individual children have a wide variety of circumstances at home (and school) to deal with. There is no cookie-cutter formula for curing depression. However, these are a few things that parents and professionals can be aware of and consider.

Trauma both present and past, can contribute to depression. A death in the family or of a loved one can affect a child's mental health and contribute to depression. Excessive time with movies and the media in general can affect the mental health of children. Violence in the media may be a contributing factor towards mental health disorders for some children, as may the quantity and type of music a child or teenager listens to. (Robertson, J., 1998). Some popular music for children can be emotionally intense, and overload on deeply emotional or intense music may affect the mood of some children and teens.

---

[34] A high sugar diet, such as is served in many school breakfasts, can contribute to diabetes.

Diet might also be a contributing factor for some childhood depression, and children do benefit from regular exercise and "fresh air". For some children and teens, love and attention are the real prescription that no drug or medicine can replace. Love is an essential element for good mental health. Talk therapy, or Interpersonal Therapy (IT), helps many children and teens to get through crises and overcome a wide variety of mental health difficulties. Cognitive behavioral therapy also is of value in treating depression and ADHD for many children, teens and adults.

Green Therapy

Richard Louv's book, *Last Child in the Woods, Saving Our Children from Nature-Deficit Disorder*, describes how children have experienced a serious decrease in the amount of time spent in natural surroundings. His book was written in an effort to help raise awareness for the positive effects that "green time" can have on children, who might otherwise become detached from the natural world. (Lugara, J., October 2004).

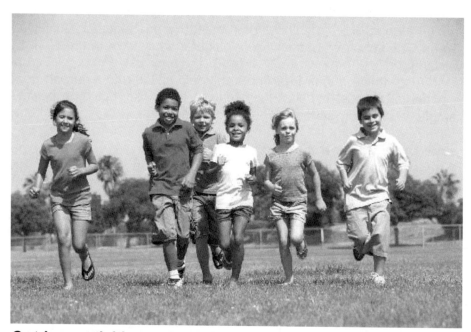

Outdoor activities and regular exercise can help children with ADHD symptoms and depression.

Psychology Today reported that children who spend time in the outdoors exercising or playing, experience a marked decrease in symptoms of

ADHD. (Psychology Today, March/April, 2006). This can be true for symptoms associated with depression also. (Heliq, 2007).

One clinical study from Duke University indicated that exercise proved to be more beneficial in treatment of mild to moderate (adult) depression than medication, in terms of both recovery and recurrence rate.[35] Further, the study indicated that exercise alone was surprisingly more efficacious in treating mild to moderate depression than medication along with exercise, both in efficacy, as well as in a reduction of recurrence rate.

The reason exercise alone may be more efficacious than exercise combined with medication, in terms of long-term recovery rates in moderate depression, might be because the mind gets used to the medication, and when you try to stop, it can leave you more vulnerable to relapses of symptoms. This can especially be the case if underlying issues have not been fully addressed.

Exercise and "Green Time"

When one teen, who had been diagnosed with ADHD, began attending the gym daily with his father, it proved to be of value to him in alleviating symptoms of ADHD. Additionally, his mother, who works in education, stated that having more structure in the household was of much value to her son. A regular, set time to eat and sleep, as well as a regular daily routine, along with daily exercise at the gym, helped her son to overcome many of the symptoms of ADHD, to the point that medication, the side effects of which were uncomfortable for her son, was no longer needed.[36]

"Green outdoor settings appear to reduce ADHD symptoms in children across a wide range of individual, residential, and case characteristics." Frances E. Kuo, PhD and Andrea Faber Taylor, PhD. September, 2004. A Potential Natural Treatment for Attention-Deficit/Hyperactivity Disorder: Evidence From a National Study. *American Journal of Public Health.* http://www.ncbi.nlm.nih.gov/pmc/articles/PMC1448497/

---

[35] Study: Exercise Has Long-Lasting Effects on Depression. September 22, 2000. Duke Today (Duke University).
[36] New Jersey Teaching Notes, 2007.

45

Exercise and "green time," as simple as walking a mile a day, has been demonstrated to be more effective in treating mild and moderate depression than medication, both in short-term and in long-term efficacy. Exercise and "green time" also can be an effective therapy for ADHD.

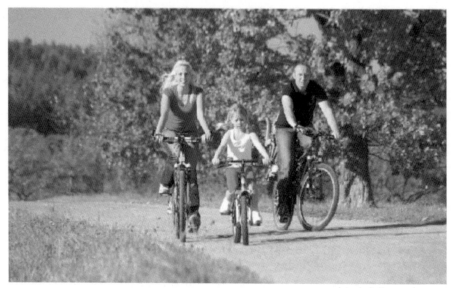

www.istoekphoto.com kzenon

Regular outdoor activities such as...

Playing in the park
Hiking
Camping
Jumping Rope
Biking
Skating
Skateboarding
Brisk Walking
Jogging

...can help children to overcome the symptoms associated with ADHD and depression.

Art Helps ADHD

Many children with symptoms of ADHD are visually-oriented. Directing that predisposition positively by parents and teachers, away from highly stimulating video games, movies and television, and rechanneling that strength towards art, can help children settle down in class and in their schoolwork.

Art can strengthen and exercise the mind, can train a child to concentrate for an extended period of time on one subject, and can provide children with a wholesome pastime that is pleasing to the eyes. Art can be likened to technology-free neurofeedback for the brain, training a child or adult in focusing and self-control. (See pages 63, 64 for information on neuro- and biofeedback).

Regular art lessons can help a child to develop a love for art and to stick with it. This can help a child to develop a longer attention span, to develop the ability to concentrate and to sit still better. Art is an important skill and therapy for children with ADHD symptoms.

Art can really make a difference. It not only helps a child to learn to concentrate, but also helps to build self-esteem, which is something that can be lacking with some children who have ADHD or other disabilities. Art can instill creativity and satisfy a child's need for visual stimulation in a gentle way, and at the same time, it can help to take the child's attention away from the TV, movies and video games, which may be part of the core reasons behind some children's inability to focus, or that may be contributing to a child's hyperactivity.

Art lessons can be an excellent investment in a child's time. Trips to art galleries are a nice outing for children. Some public schools have murals which children and teenagers have painted or are painting on the school walls in the hallways. It is an application of the use of art in the school system that is both positive and that enhances school morale. It is also a good project for children in special education, and for other children with special needs, to be involved with.

Very simply, replacing a child's TV, movie and video game time with art can contribute to improvement in ADHD symptoms.

Children who end up being labeled ADHD often are very visually-oriented. When this is channeled positively towards art, then that liability turns into a positive, with increased potential for creativity and productivity. (Barroqueira, D., 2006).

"Back then [in college] I was in fine art.
I was immersed in creating art. It helped me to be able to focus."
Ryan M., art teacher in Newark, NJ, diagnosed with ADHD in
middle school and high school.

A Few Art Resources for Children and Teens

Books:

The New Drawing on the Right Side of the Brain, 1999. *By Betty Edwards.* Great book!

Drawing With Children, 1986. *By Mona Brookes Tarher.*

Draw 50 (Animals, People, etc.)... series *By Lee J. Ames* Simple, but effective, kids love it.

Encouraging the Artist in Your Child, 1989. *By Sally Warner.*

Drawing Faces - Usborne Art Ideas, 2002. *By Jan McCafferty.*

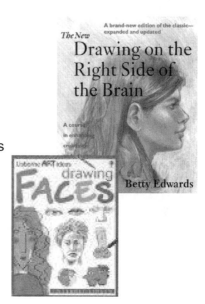

Web Sites:

Art Junction - www.artjunction.org/young.php - Art Junction is a program of the *University of Florida* and is described as a collaborative site for teachers and students. It has helpful information with details on teaching art to children, at various stages, including preschoolers, and how to nurture their creative ability, along with some specifics on what materials are best to use. It features resources for teachers, teens and children, as well as helpful links.

Something Different - www.youdraw.com is a website where you can draw your own pictures using an electronic pad on the computer, which are posted onto the site. It is something children can do so that their works get some kind of viewing audience. The images are to be published in a book, so their drawings may appear in print, which also is something positive and exciting for children. There are a number of similar sites.

Two good sites to learn to draw portraits:

About.com – Portrait Drawing
drawsketch.about.com/od/drawingportraits/Portrait_Drawing_Faces.htm

Portrait Artist.org
www.portrait-artist.org/face

Professional Art Therapy

Professional Art Therapy is a real and growing branch of mainstream (non-alternative) psychology. Art therapists are board certified and are located throughout the United States. The *American Art Therapy Association* can educate you on this non-alternative form of therapy in treating many mental health disorders in children, teens, and adults.

American Art Therapy Association (AATA).
www.arttherapy.org
The AATA represents approximately 5,000 members and 36 AATA state and regional chapters that conduct meetings and activities to promote art therapy on the local level.

Subscription Magazine Gift Ideas for Children:

- Big Backyard
- Animal Baby
- Ranger Rick

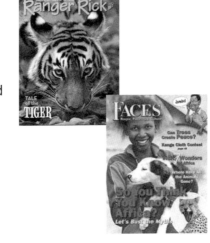

From our experience, younger and older pre-teen children look forward to every issue.

National Wildlife Federation
http://www.nwf.org
800-822-9919

- Faces Magazine
  Cobblestone & Cricket

Faces is a very colorful, interesting subscription magazine for children ages 9 to14, which teaches them about people and cultures from all over the world. www.cobblestonepub.com

Children need your time,
attention, approval and LOVE

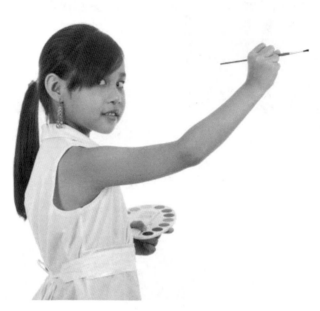

***Children and ART- A healthy mix and part of a natural "cure"
for many children and teens with ADHD***

**One of our greatest emotional and psychological needs is
love.** Without love, psychological problems are more likely to increase
or intensify. Love is a healer. Love has been described as "the best
prescription". When children who manifest symptoms of ADHD receive
extra love and attention from parents, concerned professionals, teachers,
nurses, this helps nearly all children with ADHD to make progress. The
prescription "curing" symptoms of ADHD, in many situations, is not in a
drug, but is a result of receiving extra love, nurturing and attention. Some
children are very independent, whereas others need more than the usual
attention and nurturing at certain stages of their development.

Many children who have been abused may manifest symptoms
which are diagnosed as ADHD, and a disproportional number of children
from single family homes are diagnosed with ADHD. (Neven, et al., 1997).
There may be a number of reasons for this.

Children need unconditional love as well as the approval of their
parents, teachers and others. Parents need to spend time with their

children, to help them with their homework, to establish loving but firm boundaries and to protect them from harmful influences. This takes both time and much effort. The television or the unsupervised Internet are not good babysitters for children or teens. They can be tools of "isolation and distraction,"[37] as one grade school teacher commented of her students in a letter to the parents. Another educator and special education student said of her preschool students, with concern and some frustration, "these children don't need medicine, they need patience and love."[38]

A teacher never knows what a child may be going through at home, so must try to deal with children and teenagers in their care patiently and with tolerance, as many do.

A responsible adult who is overly-critical can damage a child's self-esteem, which might contribute to problems for the child later in life. Any activities that bolster self-esteem can be part of the healing effort for children with ADHD symptoms.

Some teachers and principals are a source of security for children of all ages, and it is heartwarming to see. Parents need to be patient with children and to give them their love, attention, time and approval, which can be a challenge if raising children with special needs. The constant berating or cruelly ridiculing a child can be considered to be a form of child abuse. Children need to be reasoned with and helped to understand the hows and whys of a certain action or conduct rather than be forced or bullied.

Spiritual Needs of Children and Adolescents

Not to be overlooked are the spiritual needs of children and adolescents. There is a positive correlation between children and adolescents who feel strongly connected spiritually and good mental, and even physical health. Children and teens with a strong sense of spirituality are better able to cope with chronic illnesses and are, in general, more resilient.

Commenting on a study by pediatrician Dr. Michael Yi, of Cincinnati Children's Hospital Medical Center, and Sian Cotton, PhD, research assistant professor in the department of family medicine, University of Cincinnati *Health Line* stated, "higher levels of spiritual well-being were associated with fewer depressive symptoms and better emotional well-being," connecting "spiritual well-being" with better "mental health outcomes." (Pence, K., January 8, 2009. *UC Health Line*). Similarly, a University of British Columbia study concluded that "Children who were more spiritual were happier," and that for those children in touch with an "inner belief system," "spirituality was a significant predictor

---

[37] Booker, K. 2004. Letter, Paterson, NJ
[38] Communication, Teaching Notes, 2005, Paterson, NJ.

of happiness, even after removing the variance associated with temperament." (Harper, J., January 12, 2009. *Washington Times*).

Rather than allow children to indulge in the "dark," sinister, or even "evil" things associated with some entertainment, including some popular books for children, choose books and entertainment which teach positive values, including spiritually enriching material. Give attention to the spiritual needs of your child and teen. This can contribute to better mental health, help children and adolescents to be more resilient, and might even contribute to better physical health outcomes for some children and teens.

Avoiding overburdening yourself with guilt
Maintain a Positive and Hopeful Attitude

Parents also need to be merciful to themselves and should avoid overburdening themselves with guilt. Such thoughts as, *"What did I do wrong? Why didn't I act sooner? If only we had,"* accomplish little and only add to the burden of a parent. The decision of whether or not to use medication can be an agonizing one for many parents at times.

Guilt can wear a family down. By dealing with the present, looking forward rather than backward, and doing everything you can do now rather than dwelling on the past, you can develop a positive, forward looking attitude that is solution-oriented. If mistakes were made, it should be remembered that *"Life is all about making mistakes and learning from them."* By addressing lifestyle changes, solutions can be reached, contributing to a better state of mind for the child and family. No family, no parents and no children are perfect. We can't expect perfection of ourselves or from any of our children. We need to maintain balance and a positive attitude towards our children, especially those with special needs or less-than-perfect circumstances.

One mother whose daughter had been diagnosed with ADHD said that she had to work hard to maintain a positive attitude towards her daughter. (It wasn't her natural inclination). If we are able to do that, it will be reflected in the way we speak and treat our child, and will result in a better long-term relationship with him or her. If we believe in the children and maintain hope, commend them for anything at all positive in their progress or accomplishments, this will be reflected in our tone of voice and conduct towards the child, and the child will pick up on this. Build on the positives. This will help the child, in turn, to see themselves positively, and not to give up when difficulties arise in their life and circumstances. Problems and difficulties *will* arise in everyone's life, and by building on strengths, a child learns to be resilient. Never give up. *"Love hopes all things."*

Chapter 5

Educational Solutions
Workable Solutions from within Schools
Educational Remediation
One-on-one Attention
Specific Teaching Techniques
18 Positive Educational Ideas
Mentoring, Tutoring
Coaching, Coaching Resources
Reading
Conclusion

"Many elementary school children rated by their teacher as having clinically significant inattentive symptoms, do not show similar symptoms the following year." David Rabiner, Ph.D., of Duke University, commenting on a clinical study of children with attentional difficulties. The study was published in the *Journal of Developmental and Behavioral Pediatric,* April 2012.

"Various explanations are possible including positive changes associated with maturation, the resolution of a significant life stressor, or perhaps improved nutrition and/or sleep. Teachers may also use rating scales differently, with some teachers prone to assign higher ratings than others.

However, it is also possible for some children, a change in classroom context, is an important factor. This echoes findings obtained with middle school students, where ratings of ADHD symptoms between teachers often do not show strong agreement. The difference has been attributed by some researchers to the unique characteristics associated with different classrooms."

Workable educational solutions
from within the school system and at home

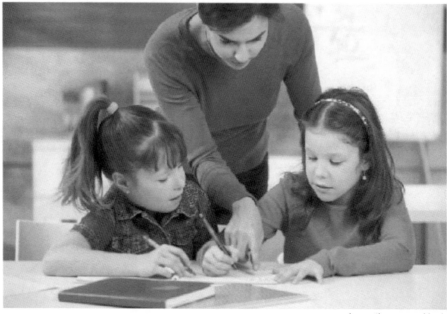

www.dreamtime.com Nyul

Educational Remediation

In addition to lifestyle changes, educational adjustments both in school and at home can help make concentration easier for many children. Susan Ashley, Ph.D., a clinical psychologist for children with many years of experience, and who works with children with special needs daily, recommends "educational remediation" along with therapy as a mainstream intervention for ADHD, rather than medication as the front-line treatment. (Ashley, S., PhD, 2005). This can result in long-term positive gains in a child's ability to focus, behave appropriately in school, and succeed in the classroom.

One-on-One Attention

Many children with learning disorders, especially those without fathers, benefit from individual one-on-one attention. Instructional assistants are available in some situations in school and this can be of help for many children.

Additionally, mentoring programs such as *Big Brother* can provide positive role models and warm encouragement. One substitute teacher in a large inner city said that what he valued most about his work was his ability to be a positive role model and father-figure to fatherless boys.

After-school tutoring to help children or teens with reading, math, or other subjects, may also be available through schools, public libraries[39] and some after-school programs, and this has also helped many to get through difficult periods in their education and to pass classes they might otherwise not have.

In the case of utilizing a reading coach after school, both the practical attention given to reading, as well as the stability and safe haven created through the one-on-one attention[40] can be stabilizing to children. A child might be totally unfocused in a classroom with 20 other children, yet might be able to focus well in a one-on-one, or small group setting.

A child might not have anyone to discuss serious issues such as divorce of their parents, and school psychologists as well as social workers and counselors can listen compassionately to children and teens. A quick amphetamine fix isn't necessarily the answer for a child who is disturbed by family issues. Qualified professionals can also support children in an Interpersonal or Talk Therapy setting. A good support team can make a huge difference.

Mentors from various programs, both educational, and through community and religious-based programs,[41] such as personal, supervised bible study, can be of help for some struggling fatherless boys and girls, as well as for some children with symptoms associated with ADHD. But especially, parents should take time to give one-on-one attention to their children.

Read with your child, take time to talk to him or her, put them to bed and read to them at night, help them regularly and patiently with their homework. Don't delegate parenting to others, but find joy in your active role as a parent, or in some cases, grandparent or guardian. Try not to expect or demand perfection, be tolerant and build on your child's strengths by giving him or her a sense of approval.

---

[39] McNuff, J., 2005. Paterson, NJ.
[40] Reading Recovery, www.readingrecovery.org.
[41] New Jersey Teaching Notes, 2005-2010.

Some specific teaching techniques that can be helpful:

Use of visual aids and pictures - Children with ADHD symptoms are often highly visual, as are many children today. One professional estimate is that 80% of today's children are visually-oriented. However, from observation it seems as if a high percentage of children who display symptoms of ADHD are "wired" visually, to a greater degree than the average child.

Break larger assignments into smaller tasks.[42] - This helps children with attentional problems to focus. Additionally, some teachers have found that seating children with attention problems, close to the teacher's desk, and within eye contact, is helpful. Careful attention to seating arrangements in general can help.

A buddy system, where progressive and well-adjusted students team up with students who have learning difficulties, has proven to be an effective way of helping the struggling student, and in teaching students who are in a position to give, to find joy and fulfillment in helping others.

"When you hear the word ADD, the next word that follows is medication. 75-80% of those who are diagnosed with ADHD will at some point be prescribed medication. "Why the push for medication? Why not urge for parent training, specialized classrooms and social skills training? We can hypothesize why parents are pressured. Medication is relatively inexpensive, highly profitable, easy to give and takes almost no effort. Parenting is a tough job. 'If a pill can make your job easier, why not?' We need to ask, 'What can I do instead?'" (condensed for brevity).
Susan Ashley, Ph.D., Clinical Psychologist - *ADD & ADHD Answer Book - The Top 275 Questions Parents Ask.*

---

[42] Some of the ideas on this page and the following pages are adapted from Sandra Rief's book, *How to Reach and Teach ADD/ADHD Children,* 1987.

18 Positive Educational Ideas
that can be of value for children with symptoms of ADHD

1. **Work with children on an individual level**, one-on-one one. Children with special needs benefit from one-on-one attention. Provide mentors, instructional assistants, and/or enroll a child in after-school tutoring or reading assistance.

2. **Clarity and structure** - Clear step-by-step instructions help children with attentional difficulties to better focus.

3. **Creative, engaging, pro-active teaching** is of importance for children with symptoms of ADHD. Some children do better orally with their schoolwork and can answer questions when they are taught, but may find it difficult to focus on written assignments and tests.

4. **School psychologists and social workers**, as part of a **support team**, can be of help. Children and young teens have a refuge where they can talk about distracting issues with other students, teachers or family, or situations that come up during the day. Social workers in the public schools and substance abuse counselors have increasingly taken on the role usually reserved for psychologists. They, also, have become a vital link for struggling children and youth. Some guidance counselors and school administrators also become part of the young student's day-to-day support team.

5. **Parental training** - Educating parents through parental training has been recommended as a part of a school effort to help children by helping the parents and family. Some public school principals have arranged for informative parental training sessions for parents of children in their school. Some local community and social programs, as well as some religious organizations also feature various forms of parental and family training. Some school principals arrange for simple instructions on the subjects of homework and media issues at home, such as violence in the media and home-Internet safety, for the parents, sent to parents for review and to sign-off on in the beginning of the school year. (Bi-lingual instructions are helpful in many communities).

6. **Open communication between school and family** is of importance. This requires effort on the part of both teachers, administrators and parents.

7. **Positive reinforcement** – While providing needed structure, limits and, at times, discipline, teachers and administrators who focus on the positive and reinforce it, build a better relationship with children and youth, and can help contribute to an academic and classroom atmosphere which helps those with attentional problems to better focus. This applies in the home environment as well.

8. **Improving one's teaching style and dedication to help children** can result in a classroom atmosphere where children with attentional difficulties can better focus. Many children with symptoms associated with ADHD need nurturing. Others need more structure. Young children are affected emotionally and psychologically from disruptions in family life such as separation or divorce, so teachers need to take these social and family issues into consideration in dealing moderately with children whose behavior is not consistent, and in making recommendations for intervention.

9. **Encourage children and teens to write regularly in a journal.** This can be an effective way to get a hold on negative emotions. Some teens find writing poetry to have an emotionally healing affect.[43]

10. **Breaking down larger tasks into smaller tasks** in the classroom can help many children with short attention spans to accomplish tasks and complete their assignments.

11. **Extensive use of graphics, color and pictures** helps all children to focus and concentrate on their schoolwork, as well as to retain more information. This is especially true of children with symptoms of ADHD.

12. **Attention to seating arrangements** in class for children with learning and attentional problems is of help for some children with learning difficulties and can be of help for the teacher. Children who have a hard time concentrating often do better sitting in the front of the classroom, close to the teacher's desk, or in a spot that is not in close proximity to their classmates. One special education teacher makes effective use of blinders that surround three sides of each desk, in his classroom of pre-teen students, when students are working on tasks requiring concentration such as math, in addition to spacing desks about two feet apart.

13. **Use of relaxing and subdued music** in class helps children to keep calm and focus. Also, some schools, and many teachers and principals,

---

[43] See the Society for Poetry Therapy. www.spt.com

58

are strict in their rules concerning iPods and cellphones with headphones in the classroom, in the halls and at school in general. Constant, intense music while a child or teen does his or her schoolwork, or in the students off-minutes, in school, on the school bus, or at home, can prove to be extremely distracting and "fragment" the mind and cognitive processes of a child or teen, making it difficult for him or her to concentrate on assignments requiring a high degree of cognitive skill. Additionally, much of the popular music that some young people in inner cities listen to, may be considered to be somewhat anti-social in its lyrics and attitude, which can contribute to disrespect towards authority, and a climate making it more difficult to maintain order, or for students to learn and focus. There is a lot going on in the headphones on either side of the student's ears.

Principals should be aware that iPod music during the school day at school, for some students, can contribute to a lower level of academic achievement and might also contribute to behavioral problems. Parents should also be aware of this. One young teen who could not focus on a difficult assignment stated the reason was the music in her head. She stated that she had been listening to the radio in her room at night, and the music was still dominating her thinking the following day in class.

14. **Regularly assigning homework** helps provide structure for children and teens after school, so that their after-school hours are spent constructively rather than otherwise. Television and video games after school can contribute to a lower level of concentration in class. One parent keeps video games away for his pre-teens and young teenagers during the school terms, and only allows them during vacation periods. Regular homework contributes to strengthening the cognitive abilities of a child and teen, as well as strengthening the ability to focus. Many grade school teachers regularly assign one to two hours of homework per day. When children regularly complete these assignments, it helps them to develop academically, as well as helping them to develop a good work ethic.

Children should have a well-organized location in the home for homework, free of distractions. The television and music should be off during their homework sessions, and some children and teens benefit from direct parental involvement with their homework.

If regularly assisting their children with their homework is overwhelming for the parent, and children need help, parents might consider hiring a tutor. If children or teens regularly say that they get no homework, parents should communicate with teachers to see if this is really the case. More often than not, most teachers assign regular homework in core subjects. Teachers should try to communicate with parents if the child isn't doing his or her homework regularly.

15. **Classroom buddies** from among excelling students can assist students who have difficulty concentrating. This has something of a positive effect in both directions, for the child who needs help, and for the child who is giving the assistance.

16. **Attentive teaching and/or classroom assistants** can be of value in both special education and in regular classrooms for children with ADHD symptoms, and for entire classrooms where there might be several students with special needs. Parents can inquire of their particular school system what is needed in order to obtain individual assistance for their child in class.

17. **Oral instructions, teaching and testing** can help some students academically. Many students excel when pro-active teaching methods are used such as question and answer, but might not do well when given a textbook reading and writing assignment. Different aptitudes and different types of learning styles can be taken into consideration when dealing with children with special needs or who have symptoms of ADHD.

18. **Keep movies out of the classroom**. Movies for entertainment, while commonly used as time-fillers in some classrooms, can be counterproductive in the long-run, especially for children with symptoms of ADHD. Some teachers and some schools sometimes use movies regularly as electronic baby-sitters.

Excessive TV and movie viewing, especially as a lifetime habit, can contribute to lazy mental and life-habits. Action cartoons can contribute to attentional difficulties for some children. Choose art over movies. Many movies today are fast-paced and many have macabre themes. It is of note that after movie-time in school, it may take some time for certain children to "wind down" and concentrate again on serious school work.[44] (This is referring to non-educational films for entertainment, in contrast to many educational videos which have much value in education.)

Movies usually develop themes and characters more deeply than television programs. The visual element of films is also usually more intense than most television programs. Children ponder over the scenes and meaning of what they have seen in movies, and many do not have the ability to "turn off the channel" in their minds. Children who have seen "scary movies" may find it difficult to concentrate in class, and some pre-teens have even been mentally distracted in class as a result of scenes and situations, which may be difficult-to-decode for children, even in movies such as Sponge Bob.

---

[44] New Jersey Teaching Notes 2005-2011.

More on Movies in School

Overdoing it with movies might be one contributing factor towards developing ADHD symptoms for some children. If anything, schools should discourage rather than encourage movies in school. This is especially in view of the fact that young children are indulging in movies of various degrees of violence, and that many popular children's movies are violent, very intense, or have scenes of violence or shocking violence. Schools can unwittingly or tacitly reinforce that life-pattern for many children, and some teachers and substitute teachers can be exceedingly liberal in the level of violence they present or allow in the classroom for children.

Many teachers, substitute teachers, and teaching assistants, as well as schools in general, use entertaining movies with marginal or no educational value as regular time-fillers. Parents should be aware of that, and might ask their children about movies they may be seeing in school.

Character education has proven to have much value in the public school system and in the classroom. One grade school teacher in Newark, NJ spends the first two days of the school year concentrating on character education lessons. This has benefits for the rest of the school year. Many classrooms have lessons, words and ideas featuring positive values and ideas posted on the walls and on posters in the school and classroom. In some schools, students paint positive quotes on the hallway and stairwell walls. This helps to create an atmosphere conducive to learning, good conduct and positive values.

The lessons to be learned from a large percentage of movies for children, however, even in the classroom, and what many children are generally watching at home, often presents the opposite message. Revenge, win at all costs, might-makes-right, or delight in other's suffering may be underlying themes. Further, fast-paced movies and cartoons, which might have scenes of violence and intensity, can contribute to ADHD symptoms for some children. Using entertainment-movies regularly in public grade schools and high schools, may be contributing to a lower quality of education in some schools.

Teaching positive life-skills such as helping young people to appreciate art for recreation and pleasure, encouraging young people and children to learn to play a musical instrument or write poetry, finding enjoyment in recreational sport, or to enjoy and appreciate the outdoors, can help a child or teen to mature emotionally and develop a positive set of values and life-habits.

Tutoring, Mentoring and Coaching

Tutoring, mentoring and coaching can prove to be of benefit for many children with symptoms of ADHD. The ADDA Association specifically recommends coaching for ADHD. Clinical studies indicate that coaching helps college students with ADHD in a number of ways. ADHD coaching is an emerging field that is coming into its own, and parents should consider coaching for middle or high school teenagers. In college, a coach can be used effectively in lieu of therapy for some students with ADHD. (University of North Carolina, 2011).

A coach is not a therapist or medical professional. A coach has been trained to help with the practical areas of life, which may be difficult to deal with for some with symptoms of ADHD. A coach is accessible during the day by phone, text or email, and helps the client stick to the treatment plan, goals, and keep organized.

Life-coaching is being used in a wide variety of contexts, while the ADHD coach specialist receives training and certification for this specialty. The cost of coaching is less than that of a therapist, and there are a number of organizations that can provide a list of qualified coaches in your area. Coaches can work in harmony with the psychologist, therapist or child study team.

Some who may not be receptive to other forms of treatment or therapies may show a positive response to coaching. Regular coaching sessions can be conducted by phone, webcam, and some coaches may work in person, or use a combination of these approaches. A coach might speak to a client daily for 15 minutes, or at other scheduled times for longer periods.

Care should be taken to choose a coach that fits into your personal style and one that both you and your teen get along with and feel comfortable with. For adults who have been diagnosed with ADHD, psychotherapy, family therapy, marital counseling and coaching, are some of the possible avenues of support. Support groups can also be of help for some adults or parents.

Coaching Resources

ADHD Coach Academy
www.addcoachacademy.com

Institute for Advancing AD/HD Coaching (IAAC)
www.adhdcoachinstitute.org

ADHD Coaches Organization
www.adhdcoaches.org

International Coach Federation (ICF)
www.coachfederation.org

Reading for Education and Pleasure

Teaching children to enjoy reading, as well as to understand what they read, is of much importance and value. Approximately 23% of adults in the United States are considered to be functionally illiterate. (Literacy. *Wisconsin Department of Public Instruction*, 2002). Children who read rather than excessively watch television, can better develop the ability to concentrate, and are better equipped for academic and future career success.[45]

One professional reading coach who has coached "hundreds" of children with ADHD symptoms, stated that "one of the greatest tragedies of this world is that children no longer know how to sit down alone and find pleasure in reading a good book." [46] Parents who are aware of that can reverse this trend with their own children. Teach your child or student to appreciate the value of reading. Reading, without the television, iPod, music or other electronic distractions, can be refreshing to the mind and soul.

> The AYCNP website features a book list with close to 200 positive books of value for children and teens. Please see: www.winmentalhealth.com/best_childrens_books.php

Neurofeedback and Biofeedback

The mind has been likened to a muscle that needs to be exercised and that can be strengthened with exercise. Neurofeedback can be likened to exercise for the mind. It can strengthen the mind and contribute to greater self-control. It is high-tech, can be costly, but some have concluded that, in reality, it is no more costly in the long-term than taking prescription stimulant medicine.

Neurofeedback involves attaching electrodes to the head, while the client works through mental exercises, which are measured to provide feedback on brain activity. Biofeeback involves regulating other parts of the body such as the skin, heart, and so on, while neurofeedback focuses only on the central nervous system.

Neurofeedback and biofeedback should only be performed professionally, after a thorough examination and by a licensed, trustworthy practicioner. While not as widely accepted as some other forms of treatment, there is evidence that neurofeedback can be effective.

---

[45] Wall Street Journal, 2007.
[46] McNuff, J., 2005. Paterson, NJ Public Library.

A child or adult can learn to develop the ability to concentrate and focus through neurofeedback, and both neuro- and biofeedback are being applied to a wide range of mental health situations and disorders, including anxiety, bipolar disorder, OCD, epilepsy, alcoholism and drug abuse.

Neurofeedback is not as mysterious as it might seem at first, and can be considered to be a way to exercise or strengthen and better control one's mind, and in the case of biofeedback, better regulate bodily functions as well. It can be used along with other forms of therapy and self-help measures.

While more research is needed, neurofeedback has become a somewhat accepted form of treatment, a more or less mainstream approach to treating ADHD and some other disorders. Clinical studies indicate that neurofeedback does result in "significant improvement" for children with ADHD using both objective and subjective (parental ratings) scales. (Lubar, J.F., et al., March 20, 1995). A meta-analysis of studies on neurofeedback for treating pediatric ADHD, published in 2011 from researchers of Ohio State University, concluded that neurofeedback is "probably efficacious". (Lofthouse, N,I,, et al., November 16, 2011).

Biofeedback/Neurofeedback Resources

The Association for Applied Physiology and Biofeedback
www.aapb.org

The International Society for Neurofeedback & Research
www.isnr.org

What is Neurofeedback?, by D. Corydon Hammond, Ph.D.
www.nhcak.com/pdfs/what%20is%20nfb.pdf

New York Biofeedback Services has good information
on the subject on its website. www.nybiofeedback.com

Chapter 6

Resources
Helpful References
Mental Health Checklist for Parents and Educators
Charts and Graphs
Bibliography
Index

Choose art over violence for better mental health for yourself and your children.

Helpful References

ADD & ADHD Question and Answer Book, *Professional Answers to 275 of the Top Questions Parents Ask.* 2005. Susan Ashley, Ph.D. Ashley is a clinical psychologist who works with children. She leans towards advocating non-pharmaceutical interventions for ADHD as a front-line strategy. Her book is an excellent resource for parents.

The ADHD Workbook for Kids: *Helping Children Gain Self-Confidence, Social Skills, and Self-Control.* 2008. Lawrence Shapiro, Ph.D.

Attention Research Update
www.helpforadd.com
email to subscribe: attentionresearchupdate@helpforadd.com

Attention Research Update is one of the most well-researched newsletters and websites on ADHD.

David Rabiner, Ph.D., Senior Research Scientist
Center for Child and Family Policy
Duke University, Durham, NC

The Antidepressant Solution: *A Step by Step Guide to Safely Overcoming Antidepressant Withdrawal, Dependence and Addiction.* 2007. Joseph Glenmullen, M.D. See also, *Prozac Backlash* by the same author.

Are We Giving Kids Too Many Drugs? *Medicating Young Minds.* November, 2003. *Time Magazine.*[47]

Bipolar Children, 2007. Edited by Sharna Olfman, Ph.D. *Bipolar Children* describes the over-diagnosis of bipolar disorder in children, the overmedicating of children who are labeled "bipolar," and some of the reasons for this. This provides excellent documentation from a number of writers on a serious issue.

Brain Exercises to Cure ADHD. 2008. Amnon Gimpel, M.D. The mind is like a muscle. By exercising it, we develop our power of concentration and can overcome certain symptoms of ADHD. Brain exercises help children strengthen the mind. Social skills and self-control can be learned and developed.

---

[47] Vincent Iannelli, M.D., author and website counselor (About.com), who sometimes supports medications for children, states, "this article does a fairly good job of describing the risks vs. benefits of treatment."

Blaming the Brain: *The Truth About Drugs and Mental Health.* 1998. Elliot Valenstein, Ph.D. *Blaming the Brain* looks at the history of psychiatric treatment, and presents evidence that mental illness is not like diabetes, high blood pressure or heart disease. Valenstein disagrees with the medical model of mental health, and the opinion that "chemical imbalances" cause mental health disorders or that pharmaceuticals can cure them. Valenstein is professor emeritus of psychology and neuroscience at Michigan State University.

Lead Poisoning - NJ Department of Community Affairs
101 South Broad St.
Trenton, NJ 08625
www.leadsafenj.org
877-DCA-LEAD
(Contact the appropriate agency in your own state if you suspect lead poisoning).

Lead poisoning, and other environmental contaminants, are a contributing factor in 2 to 10% of cases of ADHD in the United States, according to interpretation of research by Joel Nigg, Ph.D. in *What Causes ADHD?*

McGillicuddy, Tara. ADD/ADHD Coach and Consultant newsletter is worth subscribing to. Tara frequently publicizes and hosts free information broadcasts of leading authors and authorities on ADHD. http://taramcgillicuddy.com/

The Myth of the A.D.D. Child - *50 Ways to Improve Your Child's Behavior & Attention Span Without Drugs, Labels or Coercion.* 1997. Thomas Armstrong, PhD. This contains an excellent introduction describing the history of the use of psychiatric medications and some good suggestions in terms of lifestyle changes for ADHD.

Natural Prozac: *Learning to Release Your Body's Own Anti-Depressants.* 1988. Joel Robertson, Ph.D. Non-pharmaceutical self-help and lifestyle changes, as solutions for depression (and related disorders) are highlighted. This provides an excellent explanation of how chemical imbalances are related to depression, and their origins. Robertson also documents how music can influence the chemistry of the mind and contribute to mental health disorders for some. Practical ideas for overcoming depression are found in this book.

No Child Left Different, Childhood in America series. 2006. Edited by Sharna Olfman, Ph.D., Point Park University. www.pointpark.edu/def

Olfman considers issues, medications, child-rearing, ADHD, bipolar disorder, and media violence. Articles are from a number of well-known writers, doctors and experts in the field.

Parenting Children with ADHD: *10 Lessons That Medicine Cannot Teach.* 2005. Vincent J. Monastra. *American Psychological Association (APA).* One of the most popular books of this genre.

Please Don't Label My Child: *Break the Doctor-Diagnosis-Drug Cycle and Discover Safe, Effective Choices for Your Child's Emotional Health.* 2007. Scott M. Shannon, M.D. This is a balanced look at labeling children and the current psychiatric method of labeling and medicating (the medical model), a counter-viewpoint from a mainstream psychiatrist, which makes much more sense than that of the medical model. Shannon is a pediatric psychiatrist who does prescribe medication at times. *Please Don't Label My Child* contains an excellent chapter on psychiatric labeling.

Prozac Backlash: *Overcoming the Dangers of Prozac, Zoloft, Paxil, and Other Antidepressants with Safe, Effective Alternatives.* 2000. Joseph Glennmullen, M.D. (psychiatrist). *Prozac Backlash* provides useful insight as to the limitations of psychiatric medications, providing good suggestions on possible physical causes of depression, as well as addressing lifestyle changes, rather than an over-reliance on pharmaceutical medications. See also *The Antidepressant Solution.*

Reading Recovery
International organization that gives assistance to schools in tutoring reading for first-graders. www.readingrecovery.org

Remotely Controlled - *How television is damaging our lives - and what we can do about it.* 2005. Aric Sigman, Ph.D. Sigman discusses and documents how watching even moderate amounts of television can affect health and mental health, including contributing to depression in adults and children, as well as contributing to ADHD.

Rethinking ADHD, *Integrated Approaches to Helping Children at Home and at School.* 1997. Ruth Schmidt Neven, Vicki Anderson, Tim Godber. *Rethinking ADHD* provides integrated approaches to helping children at home and at school. This is one of the best books for background information on the subject. It also documents the over-prescribing of psychiatric drugs as well as social issues involved with ADHD. *Solution-oriented.*

So Sexy, So Soon, *The New Sexualized Childhood and What Parents Can Do to Protect Their Kids.* 2007. Jean Kilbourne, Ed.D., Dianne Levin, Ph.D. This book discusses, among some other issues, media and cultural influences on sexualizing children in modem society.
     Some of the media icons and influences mentioned by name in *So Sexy So Soon* are: Bratz Dolls, other sexy cartoons, Pro-wrestling Girls,

Power Puff Girls, Disney Channel, High School Musical, Spice Girls (Let Me Be Your Lover), Christina Agueleira, L'll Kim, 50-Cent, Justin Timberlake (Sexy Back), Eminem, Barbie Lingerie - My Scene Barbie, Cosmo Girl (magazine), sexy music videos, cable TV in the (child's) bedroom.

One might add also, since the *So Sexy So Soon* book was published, Miley Cyrus' *Party in the USA* video and concert, with her controversial "pole dancing," as well as the Disney-produced Cheetah Girls. Lady Gaga is referred to by one news item as "poison" for kids in a report entitled, "Has Lady Gaga Gone Too Far?" This, in response to the strong sexual content of her video, viewed mostly by teens. (Britney Spears also has been implicated in fanning the flames of sexual child abuse, with her sexy school girl outfit and sexual music in her debut CD). *70% of TV for teens has sexual content. The average teen sees 2,000 sex acts a year on TV.*

Examples of icon television/movie VIOLENCE: Mighty Morphin Power Rangers, Transformers, Star Wars, Teenage Mutant Ninja Turtles, Pro-Wrestling, Grand Theft Auto, one of the most popular video games for inner-city boys and teens (along with others), GiJo, Batman, Incredible Hulk, other superhero movies and cartoons.

Note: Even handheld video game units can be fast-paced and overly-stimulating for the minds of some pre-teen boys. In grade school, playing hand-held video game units during recess, children kill-thy-neighbor in interactive combat and indulge in pocket sized criminal activity in Grand Theft Auto during class breaks. Does this affect their behavior in class? Does it affect their ability to concentrate, their academic performance and grades, their personality? It very likely does.

What Causes ADHD? *Understanding What Goes Wrong and Why* 2006. Joel T. Nigg, Ph.D. Michigan State University. Nigg provides technical and thorough scientific insights into the subject, with this very well-documented book. Way beyond the scope of most books on ADHD, *What Causes ADHD* is a well-rounded resource on ADHD. This is a must for writers and authors on ADHD and other children's issues.

Your Child's Health: *The Parents' One-Stop Reference Guide to: Symptoms, Emergencies, Common Illnesses, Behavior Problems, and Healthy Development.* 1991. Barton D. Schmidt, M.D., F.A.A.P. *Your Child's Health* is a good general reference for parents. A couple of specific chapters also highlight dangers of violence in TV and films for children. Barton documents the mental health implications for children of the past two decades, many of whom are indulging in movies of extreme violence and sadism from as young as kindergarten.

One other book of note for parents (and educators) is**, Mommy I'm Scared: How TV and Movies Frighten Children and What Parents Can Do About It,** 1998. Joanne Cantor, Ph.D., Professor of communication at university of Wisconsin. The overall effects over time of media violence: Desensitization towards violence and towards others' suffering, imitation of violence/violent acts. Children are often exposed to violence on the television at home, and parents might not be aware of this. This is not uncommon, and a relatively low proportion of parents use parental controls on the television (or the Internet). Cantor mentions by name, as examples of commonly embraced violence in the media, Jaws (the movie), The Day After (movie), The Incredible Hulk, Batman, Goosebumps, E.T. (which can be disturbing for young children), Alfred Hitchcock's Psycho, the Wizard of Oz (as disturbing for some young children; the Wizard of Oz is also mentioned by child psychiatrist Peter Neubauer in the same context), as examples of movies and TV with violence or disturbing scenes for children. Also mentioned are the well known R-rated "Chucky," Friday the 13th, Freddy Krueger type movies, that children are regularly exposed to on cable TV and in movie theatres.

   Her book points to both problems and solutions. Part of that solution might be in education, where teachers, principals or other community educators can help parents to understand the value of protecting children from violence in its many forms.

****

A number of the books mentioned on these pages, are available for download in whole or in part on googlebooks, at no cost.

Free downloadable coloring pages for children
There are many sites on the Internet for free coloring book downloads. You can make your own coloring book for your child featuring pages on every conceivable topic, for only the cost of the paper and ink. These are just a few sites among many where you can find free coloring pages.

Coloring Book Fun has hundreds of free coloring pages for children of all ages and levels. coloringbookfun.com

RaisingOurKids.com has a good selection of printable flower coloring pages for children, some simple, some more complex.

Free Coloring Pages: Karen's Whimsey. More complex coloring pages for older or artistically-inclined children.
http://karenswhimsy.com/free-printable-coloring-pages.shtm

Able Child is a grass roots non-profit of note in the field of ADHD for parents. www.ablechild.org

ADHD & Mental Health Checklist
--------------------------------*for Parents and Educators*

Art

If a child is visually oriented, what about enrolling your children in an art program or private lessons?

Have you looked into professional art therapy?

Do you have art books available at home for your child so he or she might develop their interest in art?

Can you spend some time teaching your children to enjoy art?

Diet

Does my child eat a good breakfast every day?

If my child has breakfast at school, do I know that he or she actually eats breakfast daily?   What is he or she eating for breakfast at home or at school?

Can improvements be made in diet and nutrition? Does my child consume a lot of sugar in different forms?

Does my child consume caffeine through soda or coffee/tea?

Green Therapy & Exercise

Have I included "green time" in my child's daily or weekly schedule? Parks, walking, hiking?

Does my child get exercise at least several times a week, at other times besides at school?

Environmental Contaminants

Is lead poisoning a possibility? Other environmental contaminants?

Can I contact the local lead poisoning agency for testing if my home or apartment might be susceptible to lead or other environmental contamination?

Is my child very sensitive to additives in food?

If so, can adjustments be made in a balanced way for a more healthful diet?

Might my child or teen be experimenting with drugs or alcohol?

Education

Am I satisfied that my child is receiving the individualized attention he needs within the school system?

Do I take an active interest in his or her school work, sitting down and helping with homework after school?

Do I communicate regularly with his or her teachers?

Does the school have an after-school program to help with homework or reading?

Is there a program for free tutoring or mentoring within the school or school district?

Does the local or county library have any special programs in tutoring or reading that can be of help?

Are there provisions within the school system for a personal assistant for my child?

Have you considered, or are you in a position to volunteer in the school that your child attends?

Is there a special summer program that my child could benefit from?

Are there academies within the school district where there may be fewer children in the classroom, or where the atmosphere might better facilitate my child's special needs?

Would simply changing classrooms help my child to concentrate better in school?[48]

Social, educational, spiritual and support

Have I made any efforts for him or her for wholesome association with other children in the community, congregation, or school, or is he or she largely isolated?

Have I looked into music lessons for my child after school or on the weekends?

Have I looked into mentoring programs, especially if the child's father is absent? Some cities (such as Newark, NJ) have free mentoring programs for qualifying teens or older children.

---

[48] Journal of Developmental and Behavioral Pediatrics, April, 2012.

How much time do I spend with my child giving him/her undivided attention?

If my child is a pre-teenager, do I spend time every day or night reading with him or her?

If the child has supportive grandparents, does he or she spend time with them regularly?

Have I instilled in my child a value system, and am I providing spiritual training? Would a regular Bible study give a child needed support, or would some other form of mentoring?

What about seeking the assistance of a professional coach?
If my child needs the help of a psychologist or therapist, do I realize that medicine is an option, not a requirement?

Sexuality
In the case of a teenager or even some pre-teens, is he or she sexually active?

Might your teenager (or child) be dabbling in, or be exposed to, pornography on the Internet, television, with friends or elsewhere?[49]

Do you have parental control filtering software installed on your computer and/or on your child's cellphone,[50] if the cellphone has access to the Internet?

Discipline
Am I consistent? Do I give discipline with firm but reasonable limits? Is the discipline administered with love?

---

[49] Exposure to pornography can make it difficult for children to concentrate in school and can contribute to symptoms related to some mental health difficulties. Pornography exposure can be an issue for young children, as well as for teens.

[50] You can purchase software for parental internet control that can be installed on cell phones. Cell phones that have access to the Internet are a common mode of downloading and transmitting pornographic images for some children and teens.

Music

What music does my children or teens listen to? Is it intense or soft? How much time does he or she spend listening to music daily or weekly?

Electronics

How many hours of television does my child watch every day?

How many hours of video games does my child play daily?

How many hours of movies does my child view each week? What types of movies does he or she view? Are they calm, or are they aggressive or violent?

Is my child regularly being exposed to violence in the media? Cartoon violence? Action violence? Video game violence? Has he developed a fondness for fantasy creatures, or violent fantasies? (Armstrong, T., 1997)[51]

How many hours a day does my child spend on online social networking communities such as Facebook, and surfing the Internet?

Is he or she largely isolated from real social contacts after school? What adjustments can be made?

If a child stays late in school daily, how is he using his time there? How does he use the computer system at school after hours?

Emotional and Support

If a child has deep-rooted emotional wounds from the present or past, has he or she opened up and talked to you or to a counselor?

Is there professional support for talk therapy available in school?[52]
Would you or your family benefit from family therapy, family counseling, or a support group?

---

[51] *The Myth of the A.D.D. Child - 50 Ways of to Improve Your Child's Behavior and Attention Span Without Drugs, Labels or Coercion* by Tom Armstrong, is a good reference book on the history of ADHD and its prescription treatment.

[52] Talk therapy, or Interpersonal Therapy, is sometimes especially helpful for children and teens.

Conclusion

ADHD doesn't have to put a child's life on indefinite hold, and it doesn't necessitate a prescription. There are a wealth of ideas that parents can put into use to help their children overcome symptoms of ADHD without medication. A combination of a number of different methods that fit into your lifestyle and resources can be effective in helping children overcome ADHD.

Children can be helped in a balanced way, without having to resort to drugs, and many have done just that. Before trying medication, first try natural methods such as lifestyle changes, to see if it doesn't make a significant difference in your child's symptoms.

Give your child extra time and attention through the most difficult years of his or her life. Give attention to your child's spiritual needs. Try to build up your child's interest in art, rather than in aggressive video games, action movies and hours alone on the Internet. If your child is musically inclined, enroll him or her in music lessons, teach your children to play a musical instrument. It is a skill that will bring enjoyment to your child for a lifetime. Try to direct your child's interest in music in a positive way. Know what they are listening to, and teach them to choose music wisely. Keep them away from intense or negative music.

Teach your child from young to love books. Reading strengthens the mind. Keep the television, video games and computer out of the child's bedroom. *A reader is a leader.*

Evaluate your child's diet, and make sure that they are getting three good meals a day, as well as healthy snacks. Pre-teen and teen girls, especially, need to eat a regular and healthy breakfast and lunch for good mental health. Spend time with your child outdoors, playing in the park, running, walking, hiking.

See what works for your child. Follow your instinct, what you feel might be causing symptoms of ADHD, and address the issues. No one formula provides the answer for every child, so take positive steps one at a time, and note where you see an improvement.

Good mental health is hard work, and it takes diligence, but the benefits are enormous. We hope that what is presented in this book helps you along the way. Continue to do careful research, put what you learn into practice, and your child will most likely be helped to overcome ADHD.

"Turn off the TV, so that in reading, you may better be!"
Encouragement from children of Paterson, NJ

TEAMS - Research-proven, non-pharmaceutical neuro-cognitive training that helps preschool children with ADHD

A 2012 clinical study with preschool children with ADHD, conducted by researchers from Queens College, NY has concluded that, *"consistently engaging children with ADHD in activities that challenge and exercise particular neurocognitive functions can strengthen the underlying neural activity that support these functions and thereby diminish ADHD symptoms."* The approach is referred to as TEAMS, which stands for, Training Executive, Attention, and Motor Skills. Activities enjoyable for children with their parents are used, which include activities of increasing difficulty designed to promote working memory, fine motor control and planning and organizational abilities. This is combined with extensive parental education about ADHD symptoms and associated problems.

The idea behind this research-proven program is *"to develop better brain function in kids,"* at an early age. About the study published in the March 5, 2012 *Journal of Attention Disorders*, David Rabiner, PhD, states, *"I found this to be one of the most interesting studies I have read during the past 10 years"*

Sources:
1. Queens College targets ADHD in pre-schoolers. (2009, Sep 24). *Queens Chronicle.*

2. Rabiner, D. (April, 2012). *Attention Research Update.*

3. Training executive attention and motor skills: A proof-of-concept study in preschool children with ADHD. *Journal of Attention Disorders*, March 15, 2012. March 5, 2012 (online). DOI: 10.1177/1087054711435681.

Further Reading and Research

1. The Art of Embracing ADHD
by Daniella Barroqueira, Illinois State University

2. Art Helps ADHD - *Inspirational experience of a grade and middle school teacher, Newark, NJ*

3. Children's television impacts executive function (EF) and contributes to later attention problems. Synopsis of research from *University of Virginia*

4. Time listening to popular music correlated with Major Depressive Disorder in adolescents, largely from *University of Pittsburgh* research

5. Music and iPod school policies

6. ISU study finds TV viewing, video game play contribute to kids' attention problems, *Iowa State University*

7. ISU study proves conclusively that violent video game play makes more aggressive kids*, Iowa State University*

8. Adjusting to Attention Deficit Disorder in adulthood, *David Rabiner, Duke University*

9. ADHD/ADD and Depression, *David Rabiner, Duke University*

10. Bipolar disorder over-diagnosed by 50%

11. FDA Alert – Liver injury risk and market withdrawal

12. Ritalin (methylphenidate) and Question of Increased Risk of Liver Cancer

The Art of Embracing ADHD
By Daniella R. Barroqueiro. Ph.D.
Associate Professor of Art Education, Illinois State University

When talking about ADHD, it is common to focus on the "downside" of the disorder, the challenges, the frustration, how to "fix" a problem or a set of problems. Notice I refer to a downside, which implies that there is also an upside to having ADHD. Intelligence, creativity, spontaneity and the ability to hyper-focus (yes, hyper-focus) are among the characteristics commonly found in people with ADHD.

Understandably, these assets are often framed in the negative because the person's ADHD is not working for them, but against them. Without a diagnosis, an awareness or knowledge of the disorder, and/or behavior modifications, these assets are obscured by the numerous liabilities of the condition. For example:

Intelligence: "She is intelligent; her test scores are high, but she is not working to her potential. She is an underachiever."

Creativity: "He has a creative energy but never seems to complete anything, so he has little to show for it."

Spontaneity: "He is so spontaneous; he just flies by the seat of his pants. He doesn't seem to know how to plan ahead or follow a schedule."

Hyper-focus: "She is so obsessed with _____ that she doesn't get any of her work done. (Fill in the blank.)"

As an art educator with ADHD, I have been both a student with ADHD and a teacher of students with ADHD. I have heard some of these things said about me, and I have said some of these things about my students. In the public schools (and at the college level), the art room is often the one place where those with ADHD feel at home. Of course, there are many students who have little interest in art making, but I believe there is something to be learned from the art education model.

The inherent subjectivity of the discipline allows for more flexibility in the way lessons are taught and in the way students interpret assignments. Even in teacher-directed projects there is often room (or at least there should be) for the self-expression of each individual student. Many lessons are necessarily restrictive in the sense that they focus on teaching a particular technique or deal with a specific subject or theme, but even in these types of lessons there are usually opportunities for students with ADHD to attend to their particular interests or their idiosyncratic ways of working, which in turn helps them to stay focused on the task at hand. Strictly speaking, there is no one right or wrong way to paint or to sculpt something.

The point is that when those with ADHD find (or create) an environment supportive to their needs, then ADHD becomes a non-issue, and in some cases, an asset. The trick is to figure out how to find or create that environment. It is my belief that when people with ADHD have taken the time to learn about ADHD in general and their own "custom brand" of ADHD in particular, they have taken the first step. Once they have begun the process of minimizing their liabilities, harnessing their creative energy and finding a productive outlet for their intelligence and hyper-focus, the possibilities are endless. The potential for success and the enjoyment of life is enormous!

Remember there are two sides to every coin. It is one thing to accept you have ADHD, but it is another to embrace it. To those with ADHD, I recommend flipping the coin and embracing what you find on the other side. I'll bet it looks a lot like intelligence, creativity, spontaneity and the ability to focus on things that matter not only to you, but also to the rest of the world.

Reprinted with kind permission from Daniella Barroqueiro, Ph.D.

Art Helps ADHD
Inspirational Experience of Grade and Middle School Teacher, Newark, NJ

Ryan M. is an art teacher in one of the most difficult grade/middle schools in Newark, NJ. He has been teaching there for a number of years and has a good rapport with the students. He is difficult to frazzle, and students request to work in his class during their breaks. He rides his bike to work for exercise, and samples of his art work, along with the work of his students, align the walls of his classroom. He creates some striking landscapes in vibrant colors.

Mr. M. describes his personality growing up as antsy and hyperactive. He was diagnosed with ADHD as a young teen and prescribed Ritalin at first, then Adderall from middle school years through high school. However, he did not like to take the medication because of the strong side effects. He didn't like the way it made him feel, and he felt that the medication contributed to a rage inside of him that was difficult to deal with.

When he graduated high school, he took up art in college, something he always enjoyed doing. He stopped taking the stimulant medications, graduated college and became an art teacher. He continues to work on his own art projects after school, but has no noticeable issues with hyperactivity or inattention. He is well-adjusted and an asset to the school, contributing to the success and development of the children he works with.

He said that there were only two things that helped him with his ADHD symptoms during his school years, playing soccer and art. He doesn't play so much soccer now, but he continues to work with art. His experience is so similar to that of Professor Barroqueiro, that it is worth mentioning here and may be an encouragement for some parents, to consider directing their children towards art, if they are struggling with attentional problems or hyperactivity.

Mr. M. states that art in school helped him to focus, the soccer helped him to find an outlet for hyperactivity. The combination worked, and his hyperfocus turned out to be an asset as an enthusiastic art teacher.

Synopsis: Children's Entertainment Television [such as Sponge Bob] **Impacts Children's Executive Function and Contributes to Later Attention Problems**

--------------------------------------*Drawing Helps Kids to Focus*

Information from University of Virginia researchers

In a study entitled, **The Immediate Impact of Different Types of Television on Young Children's Executive Function by professor** Angeline S. Lillard, PhD, and Jennifer Peterson, BA of the *Department of Psychology at the University of Virginia, Charlottesville, Virginia, researchers concluded that children's television can have a marked affect on attention problems. The paper, published September 12, 2011 in Pediatrics, states that "Previous study results have suggested a longitudinal association between entertainment television and later attention problems."*

What this study adds is, *"Using a controlled experimental design, this study found that preschool aged children were significantly impaired in executive function immediately after watching just 9 minutes of a popular fast-paced television show [Sponge Bob], relative to, after watching educational television or drawing."*

This study concludes what most of us could discern intuitively, that Sponge Bob, and other fast-paced cartoons, does indeed wind up the spring of children and can affect the attention and ability to concentrate in young children. In this study, sixty four-year-old preschool children were assigned to watch a fast-paced television cartoon, a realistic educational cartoon or to draw for nine minutes.

The children who were assigned to watch the educational cartoon and the children who were assigned to draw, performed significantly better in executive function tasks than those who watched the fast-paced cartoon.

The study states that "Parents should be aware that fast-paced television shows could at least temporarily impair young children's executive function."

Functions associated with the Executive Function (EF) are part of the skill functions associated with the prefrontal cortex, which include, goal-directed behavior, attention, working memory, inhibitory control, problem solving, self-regulation and delay of gratification (as opposed to instant gratification, commonly associated with television). EF is recognized as a key to "positive social and cognitive functioning." Therefore, EF has a bearing on the overall success of children in school, on a wide range of fronts. Long-term effects of watching television for children have been documented in some studies, this was the first to consider short-term effects. The study states that "even adults report feeling less alert immediately after watching television." And that "Entertainment television is particularly associated with long-term attention problems."

Sesame Street upped the pace of television for children, starting around 1968/1969, however, Sesame Street today is double the pace of Sesame Street when it began over 30 years ago, states Lillard and Peterson.

In addition to the fast pace of the cartoon, the authors hypothesize that the "onslaught of fantastical events," portrayed in the cartoon shown to the children in this study, may have further exacerbated the Executive Function of the children. Additionally, the study does not make conclusions about the long-term effects of watching fast-paced television, and because the cartoon segments were only nine minutes, compared to longer periods of time typically involved with television cartoons for children, the actual effects on EF, including attention, may actually be "more detrimental" than the study indicates.

The authors state that "Children watch a great deal of television," which "has been associated with long-term," and in the case of this study, "short-term," attentional problems.

****

Further information on Executive Function: Kaplan S, Berman M. Directed attention as a common resource for executive functioning and self-regulation. *Perspectives Psychology Sci*ence, 2010;5(1):43.

The Immediate Impact of Different Types of Television on Young Children's Executive Function. Angeline, S., Lilliard and Jennifer Peterson. *Pediatrics*; originally published online September 12, 2011; DOI:10.1542/peds.2010-1919
http://pediatrics.aappublications.org/content/early/2011/09/08/peds.2010-1919.full.pdf

Time Listening to Popular Music Correlated with Major Depression - *Major Depressive Disorder (MDD)* - in Adolescents - *Reading Books Helps with Major Depression in Teens*

Researchers at the University of Pittsburgh concluded that there is a correlation between Major Depression and the amount of time an adolescent spends with popular music. Conversely, Major Depression is negatively, or reversely correlated with reading print media such as books.

The study, published in the Archives of Pediatric and Adolescent Medicine, April, 2011, examined data collected through telephone interviews. During an eight-week period involving one-hundred six adolescents. The study was part of a larger neurobehavioral study of depression that was conducted between 2003 and 2008.

For each increasing quartile of audio/music use, there was an 80% increase in the odds of having Major Depression (MDD). For time spent reading, there was a 50% decrease in the odds of having MDD.

The study does not necessarily conclude a direct cause and effect relationship, although that might be one valid conclusion. Rather, there might be other correlational factors to consider in evaluating this evidence. Perhaps those who are more inclined towards music are also more inclined towards major depression. Perhaps those with major depression seek solace and solitude in music.

In any case, there seems to be strong evidence that for adolescents, there is a correlation between time spent listening to popular music and depression. This can provide encouragement for parents, educators and mental health professionals to help children and adolescents spend less time listening to popular music and more time reading.

Music and iPod* (or other music-listening devices)
--- and School Policies

Many schools have a difficult time keeping the use of electronic devices in school and in the classroom under control. One vice-principal in a city grammar and middle school declared that the administration was waging a "war on electronic devices" in school, similar to the "war on drugs" from a previous decade. She said that "we know that we won't completely win this war, but we'll keep trying."

In the International Grammar School in Sydney, Australia, the administration outright banned iPods, "the gadget of choice" in school. (An iPod can hold up to 10,000 songs, although most students might have only one or two-hundred at any one time). Not all students concurred, stating that listening to music while doing school work helped them to concentrate. However, the school administration disagreed referring to iPods and similar devices as contributing to "social isolation," The executive director of the Association of Independent Schools, Geoff Newcombe stated that iPods in school "distract students, impede their safety and stop them from communicating with classmates."

Many teachers, however, downplay the issue and allow students to listen to iPods in class, especially if students are quiet and do their work.

One of the problems, though, with use of electronics in school is, as one Newark High School Graphic Arts teacher stated, "give them an inch and they take a mile". It can be very difficult to keep electronic devices under control once they are in the school, and when there may be inconsistent or loosely enforced guidelines. Both teachers and administration get worn out with the issue, and as the school year progresses, use of electronics can get out of hand. It can contribute to needless situations with teachers in the classroom, using up teacher's time and energy dealing with the situation, and can possibly contribute to a lower quality in the academic level of individual schools.

In Barringer Preparatory High School in Newark, New Jersey, iPods and other electronic devices are banned in school. Not an iPod (or their equivalents) can be seen in the hallways, and students attempting to bring them in, get stopped at the entrance metal detectors, and are required to turn in their electronics at the door before coming into the school. They can then collect their devices at the end of the day, a rather humane antidote to a problem that perplexes some school systems.

---

* iPod is tradename of Apple, and is used here in a generic sense for iPods and similar music-listening devices. Many students simply use headphones with their cellphone for listening to music in school.

Students seem to have no issue with the no ipod/cellphone policy, in fact, Barringer Prep is a good example of a school, in a difficult area of Newark to teach in, where there is good order in the hallways, where security guards have good control and a good rapport with students, and where there is a sparcity of hallway-related security issues.

Reference: No more songs in their pockets: School bans iPods. By Linda Doherty and Jordan Baker. *The Sydney Morning Herald.*

****

ISU study finds TV viewing, video game play contribute to kids' attention problems
Reprinted with permission from Iowa State University public relations website.

AMES, Iowa - Parents looking to get their kid's attention - or keeping them focused at home and in the classroom - should try to limit their television viewing and video game play. That's because a new study led by three Iowa State University psychologists has found that both viewing television and playing video games are associated with increased attention problems in youths.

The research, which included both elementary school-age and college-age participants, found that children who exceeded the two hours per day of screen time recommended by the American Academy of Pediatrics were 1.5 to 2 times more likely to be above average in attention problems.

"There isn't an exact number of hours when screen time contributes to attention problems, but the AAP recommendation of no more than two hours a day provides a good reference point," said Edward Swing, an Iowa State psychology doctoral candidate and lead researcher in the study. "Most children are way above that. In our sample, children's total average time with television and video games is 4.26 hours per day, which is actually low compared to the national average."

Collaborating with Swing on the research were ISU's Douglas Gentile, an associate professor of psychology and Craig Anderson, a Distinguished Professor of psychology; and David Walsh, a Minneapolis psychologist. Their study will be published in the August print issue of Pediatrics -- the journal of the American Academy of Pediatrics.

Studies on elementary, college-aged youths
The researchers assessed 1,323 children in third, fourth and fifth grades over 13 months, using reports from the parents and children about their

video game and television habits, as well as teacher reports of attention problems. Another group of 210 college students provided self-reports of television habits, video game exposure and attention problems.

Previous research had associated television viewing with attention problems in children. The new study also found similar effects from the amount of time spent with video games.

"It is still not clear why screen media may increase attention problems, but many researchers speculate that it may be due to rapid-pacing, or the natural attention grabbing aspects that television and video games use," Swing said. Gentile reports that the pace of television programming has been quickened by "the MTV effect."

"When MTV came on, it started showing music videos that had very quick edits -- cuts once every second or two," Gentile said. "Consequently, the pacing of other television and films sped up too, with much quicker edits." He says that quicker pace may have some brain-changing effects when it comes to attention span. "Brain science demonstrates that the brain becomes what the brain does," Gentile said. "If we train the brain to require constant stimulation and constant flickering lights, changes in sound and camera angle, or immediate feedback, such as video games can provide, then when the child lands in the classroom where the teacher doesn't have a million-dollar-per-episode budget, it may be hard to get children to sustain their attention." The study showed that the effect was similar in magnitude between video games and TV viewing.

TV, video games may contribute to ADHD

Based on the study's findings, Swing and Gentile conclude that TV and video game viewing may be one contributing factor for attention deficit hyperactivity disorder (ADHD) in children.

"ADHD is a medical condition, but it's a brain condition," Gentile said. "We know that the brain adapts and changes based on the environmental stimuli to which it is exposed repeatedly. Therefore, it is not unreasonable to believe that environmental stimuli can increase the risk for a medical condition like ADHD in the same way that environmental stimuli, like cigarettes, can increase the risk for cancer."

"Although we did not specifically study the medical condition of ADHD in these studies, we did focus on the kinds of attention problems that are experienced by students with ADHD," added Swing. "We were surprised, for example, that attention problems in the classroom would increase in just one year for those children with the highest screen time."

ISU study proves conclusively that violent video game play makes more aggressive kids

Reprinted with permission from Iowa State University public relations website.

AMES, Iowa -- Iowa State University Distinguished Professor of Psychology Craig Anderson has made much of his life's work studying how violent video game play affects youth behavior. And he says a new study he led, analyzing 130 research reports on more than 130,000 subjects worldwide, proves conclusively that exposure to violent video games makes more aggressive, less caring kids -- regardless of their age, sex or culture.

The study was published today in the March 2010 issue of the Psychological Bulletin, an American Psychological Association journal. It reports that exposure to violent video games is a causal risk factor for increased aggressive thoughts and behavior, and decreased empathy and prosocial behavior in youths.

"We can now say with utmost confidence that regardless of research method -- that is experimental, correlational, or longitudinal -- and regardless of the cultures tested in this study [East and West], you get the same effects," said Anderson, who is also director of Iowa State's Center for the Study of Violence. "And the effects are that exposure to violent video games increases the likelihood of aggressive behavior in both short-term and long-term contexts. Such exposure also increases aggressive thinking and aggressive affect, and decreases prosocial behavior."

The study was conducted by a team of eight researchers, including ISU psychology graduate students Edward Swing and Muniba Saleem; and Brad Bushman, a former Iowa State psychology professor who now is on the faculty at the University of Michigan. Also on the team were the top video game researchers from Japan - Akiko Shibuya from Keio University and Nobuko Ihori from Ochanomizu University - and Hannah Rothstein, a noted scholar on meta-analytic review from the City University of New York.

The following (pages 88 to 92) is reprinted from *Attention Research Update* with permission from David Rabiner, Ph.D., Director of Undergraduate Studies. Dept. of Psychology & Neuroscience. Senior Research Scientist. Center for Child and Family Policy. Duke University.

Adjusting to Attention Deficit Disorder in adulthood

On the positive side, approximately one third of children with ADHD/ADD appear to be relatively well adjusted and symptom free as young adults. Although reliable predictors of such good adult outcome have not been fully identified there are several factors that are important to note.

First, not surprisingly, higher levels of intellectual functioning and better school performance are associated with better outcomes. Second, the absence of severe behavior and conduct problems during childhood, particularly before age 10, is associated with better adult outcome. And finally, children with ADHD/ADD who manage to get along well with their peers are likely to have better adjustments as adults.

These factors have clear implications for parents. It is very important to stress that it does not appear to be the primary symptoms of ADHD/ADD - inattention, hyperactivity, and impulsivity - that are most directly responsible for the negative adult outcomes that many children with ADHD/ADD attain. Instead, it is the behavioral, social, and academic difficulties that children with ADHD/ADD are at increased risk for that may be most clearly linked to negative adult outcome.

What this means is that if parents can succeed in preventing the development of these secondary problems - i.e. academic struggles, social problems, severe behavioral problems - their child is likely to have a much more successful adjustment in adolescence and young adulthood. Carefully monitoring a child's overall development, and not just focusing on ADHD/ADD symptoms, is thus critically important. When academic, behavioral, and social difficulties arise, working hard to address these problems is of paramount importance.

Medication Treatment for ADHD

What other interventions have already been tried?
Some children with ADHD can have their symptoms effectively managed via other means including appropriate behavioral and educational interventions. If you are concerned about using medication with your child, make sure that non-medical interventions have been tried first. This is an important issue to discuss with your child's physician…

How much difficulty are my child's symptoms actually creating?
The degree of impairment in academic, social, and behavioral functioning caused by ADHD can vary substantially. If the impairment experienced by your child is on the modest side, medication can be less essential than when the impairment is great.

What is my child's attitude toward taking medication?
It is very important to discuss the rational for using medication with the child. The child needs to know why it is being suggested and how it can be helpful. This is especially true for older children and adolescents, who may have concerns about being teased should their peers find out that they are taking medicine. If children have strong objections to taking medication, these should be discussed and understood. Should these objections persist, using medication my not be productive.

Will objective information about the effects of medication be provided?
In my opinion, this is critical. Despite the well documented benefits of stimulant medication, as many as 20-30% of children do not experience significant benefits. In addition, many parents are surprised to learn that when children with ADHD receive only a placebo (i.e. medication that appears to be the real thing but is not), teachers frequently report significant improvement in the child's behavior. This means that some children may receive stimulant medication for a sustained period even though they derive no objective benefit from it.

What causes this placebo effect? No one knows for sure, but when teachers are aware that a child has started medication, it is difficult for them to provide an objective, unbiased account of the child's behavior. Some children may also do better when they believe they are receiving medication that is supposed to help. This can make it difficult for parents and physicians to get objective information to use in making decisions about long term medication use.

Despite the placebo effect noted above, there are many children for whom the response is so dramatic that it seems impossible to attribute the improvement to a simple placebo response. Studies have found, however, that sometimes the improvement reported when a child is receiving placebo can also be quite dramatic. In addition, determining the optimum dose for a child in the absence of receiving objective feedback is also difficult. *End quote/article*

Dr. Rabiner then describes a method by which parents, along with teachers, can test whether or not medication is actually affecting a positive response or if there are other factors that are mainly responsible.

See: Medication Treatment for ADHD, David Rabiner, Ph.D.
Attention Research Update newsletter.
http://www.helpforadd.com/medical-treatment

****

ADHD/ADD and Depression

Several well-conducted studies have shown that children with Attention Deficit Hyperactivity Disorder/Attention Deficit Disorder, are more likely than others to become depressed at some time during their development. In fact, their risk for developing depression is as much as 3 times greater than for other children.

What does depression look like in a child?

What, then, would a "typical" depressed child look like? Although there of course would be wide variations from child to child, such a child might seem to be extremely irritable and/or very sad, and this would represent a distinct change from their typical state. They might stop participating or getting excited about things they used to enjoy and display a distinct change in eating patterns. You would notice them as being less energetic, they might complain about being unable to sleep well, and they might start referring to themselves in critical and disparaging ways. It is also quite common for school grades to suffer as their concentration is impaired, as does their energy devoted to any task. As noted above, this pattern of behavior would persist for at least several weeks, and would appear as a real change in how the child typically is. (It is also important to note, however, that some children can experience a chronic, somewhat less intense type of mood disorder that is called dysthymic disorder. In this disorder, there is a pervasive and ongoing pattern of depressed mood rather than a more distinct change from the child's typical way of appearing).

Depression and Children with Attention Deficit Hyperactivity Disorder/Attention Deficit Disorder

As noted above, children with ADHD/ADD appear to be at increased risk for the development of depression. In addition, it is important to recognize that in some children, the symptoms of depression can be incorrectly diagnosed as reflecting ADHD/ADD. That is because diminished concentration, failing to complete tasks, and even agitated

90

behavior that can resemble hyperactive symptoms can often be found in children who are depressed. It is thus quite important to be certain that depression has been ruled out as an explanation for the symptoms of ADHD/ADD a child may be displaying. Having said this, please remember that for many children, Attention Deficit Hyperactivity Disorder/Attention Deficit Disorder and depression can co-occur - i.e. be present at the same time. Thus, it is not always a matter of ruling out depression to diagnose ADHD/ADD, or ruling out ADHD/ADD and diagnosing depression. This is because in some situations both diagnoses would be appropriate and is one of the reasons why a careful evaluation by a trained child mental health professional can be so important to have done.

Recent research has suggested that in children with ADHD/ADD who are depressed, the depression is not simply the result of demoralization that can result from the day to day struggles that having ADHD/ADD can cause. Instead, although such struggles may be an important risk factor that makes the development of depression in children with Attention Deficit Hyperactivity Disorder/Attention Deficit Disorder more likely, depression in children with ADHD/ADD is often a distinct disorder and not merely "demoralization".

The results of one recent study indicated that the strongest predictor of persistent major depression in children with ADHD/ADD was interpersonal difficulties (i.e. being unable to get along well with peers). In contrast, school difficulty and severity of Attention Deficit Hyperactivity Disorder/Attention Deficit Disorder symptoms were not associated with persistent major depression. In addition, the marked diminishment of ADHD/ADD symptoms did not necessarily predict a corresponding remission of depressive symptoms. In other words, the course of ADHD/ADD symptoms and the course of depressive symptoms in this sample of children appeared to be relatively distinct.

Implications

Depression in children can be effectively treated with psychological intervention. In fact, the evidence to support the efficacy of psychological interventions for depression in children and adolescents is currently more compelling than the evidence supporting the use of medication.

The important point that can be taken from this study, I think, is that parents need to be sensitive to recognizing the symptoms of depression in their child, and not to simply assume that it is just another facet of their child's ADHD/ADD. In addition, if a child with ADHD/ADD does develop depression as well, treatments that target the depressive symptoms specifically need to be implemented. As this study shows, one should not assume that just addressing the difficulties caused by the Attention Deficit Hyperactivity Disorder/Attention Deficit Disorder symptoms will also alleviate a child's depression.

If you have concerns about depression in your child, a thorough evaluation by an experienced child mental health professional is strongly recommended. This can be a difficult diagnosis to correctly make in children, and you really want to be dealing with someone who has extensive experience in this area.

Articles reprinted with permission From David Rabiner
Article from *ADHD/ADD and Depression*
www.helpforadd.com/depression-with-add

David Rabiner, Ph.D.
Director of Undergraduate Studies
Dept. of Psychology & Neuroscience
Senior Research Scientist
Center for Child and Family Policy
Duke University

****

Bipolar Disorder Over-diagnosed by 50%

Using a self-administered questionnaire, Structured Clinical Interview for DSM-IV (SCID) and a review of the family history, the research team found that "fewer than half of the patients diagnosed with bipolar disorder, actually met the criteria for this condition, based on the SCID diagnostic questionnaire. (M. Zimmerman, M.D., at Brown Medical School).

In July 2009 a study of 82 patients previously (erroneously) diagnosed with bipolar disorder revealed that the vast majority - 68 of the 82 (82.9%) - had major depression. The majority of the others had eating disorders, anxiety disorders, borderline personality disorder, impulse control disorders, and other disorders, rather than bipolar disorder, according to the DSM-IV (SCID) test. Bipolar disorder "is typically treated with mood-stabilizing drugs that can have side effects - including effects on the kidneys, liver, and metabolic and immune systems, and means some patients are likely not getting the appropriate care for the problems they do have."

"The results of this study suggest that bipolar disorder is being over-diagnosed," Zimmerman says. Such instances are cause for significant concern given the serious side effects of mood stabilizing drugs - the standard treatment for bipolar disorder, which include possible impact to renal, endocrine, hepatic, immunologic, and metabolic function. Patients and physicians are both susceptible to the misdiagnosis. Some patients "are looking for a magic pill that will cure all ills," Zimmerman told the Providence Journal, as a way to skirt the difficult work of psychotherapy.

Sources: biomed.brown.edu/facultyupdate/news.php
www.winmentalhealth.com/bipolar.disorder.overdiagnosed.php

****

Possible Potential for Liver Damage

Some parents have expressed concern over potential liver damage from use of stimulant medications. While there is no proof that stimulant medications at large cause liver damage, the long-term effects of psychiatric medications in general, including stimulant medications, has not been studied to a significant extent. Therefore, the question still remains, what are the long-term physical effects of the use of psychiatric medications on children and teens? The following is one FDA alert concerning the stimulant medication pemoline.

****

FDA ALERT: Liver Injury Risk and Market Withdrawal (October, 2005).

The Federal Drug Administration has concluded that the overall liver toxicity from Cylert and generic pemoline products outweighs the benefits of this drug. In May 2005, Abbott chose to stop sales and marketing of Cylert in the U.S. All generic companies have also agreed to stop sales and marketing of this product in the U.S. (pemoline tablets and chewable tablets). Cylert is a central nervous system stimulant indicated for the treatment of Attention Deficit Hyperactivity Disorder (ADHD). This product is considered second-line therapy for ADHD, because of its association with life-threatening hepatic failure (see BOX WARNING in product label and patient package insert).

****

Ritalin (methylphenidate) and Question of Increased Risk of Liver Cancer

A serious issue that has been the subject of study is, does stimulant medication use among children and teens contribute to a higher rate to cancer? At present, this is an undetermined question. There has been one study involving 12 children with ADHD, conducted by the *University of Texas M.D. Anderson Cancer Center in Houston* and the *University of Texas Medical Branch at Galveston,* 2005, which concluded that chromosome damage, thought to be a precursor to the development of cancer, occurred at three-times the normal rate in eight-year olds who took Ritalin (methylphenidate) over a three-month period. [1]

Lead researcher Randa A. El-Zein, MD, PhD, states*, "It was pretty surprising to me that all of the children taking [Ritalin] showed an increase in chromosome abnormalities in a relatively short period of time."* Toxicologist and senior investigator of the study, Marvin Legator, PhD, states, *"Nobody is saying that because a child takes Ritalin he or she will develop cancer. There is nothing certain about this yet, but this is potentially a very large risk factor."*

A study from 1993 indicated that mice given Ritalin at a similar proportional level as would be given to children, developed liver tumors, including malignant cancers The *Cancer Prevention Coalition,* a Chicago based 501 (c)3 non-profit states,

"The National Toxicology Program accepted responsibility for conducting trials on carcinogenicity and in June 1993 released results showing that feeding mice Ritalin induced liver tumors including very rare and highly malignant cancers. These results were found at levels close to those routinely prescribed for children." The *Cancer Prevention Coalition* was founded by Samuel S. Epstein, M.D., Professor emeritus Environmental & Occupational Medicine, University of Illinois, Chicago. [2]

The above referenced study concluded in the Pathology Findings section, "The principal lesions associated with the administration of methylphenidate hydrochloride occurred in the liver." [3]

Types of abnormalities consisted of **Eosinophilic foci**,[3] which consist of cells that tend to be larger than adjacent normal hepatocytes with eosinophilia due to increased cytoplasmic mitochondria and/or smooth endoplasmic reticulum [4] (cytolplasmic mitochondria and endoplasmic reticulum are organelles within the cell). "Increased incidences of **hepatoblastoma**," [3] which is the most common liver cancer in children. [4] Also, "Increased incidences of **hepatocellular adenoma**," [3] were noted. [3] Hepatocellular adenomas (HAs) are also known as hepatic adenomas or liver cell adenomas. They are rare, benign tumors… [4]

Despite the above research, more research would be necessary to come to definite conclusions about a possible strong link between methylphenidate or other stimulant drugs, and cancer. It is a possibility, but there is not yet enough direct scientific evidence for such a conclusion.

References for Ritalin (methylphenidate) and liver cancer

1. Does Ritalin Increase Cancer Risk in Children? Small Study Suggests Possible Chromosome Damage, but Some Experts Skeptical, March 1, 2005. Salynn Boyles. *WebMD Health News.*

2. Ritalin: Stimulant for Cancer. Epstein, M.D., Samuel S. *Cancer Prevent Coalition.* Chicago, Illinois. Retrieved March 7, 2012.
http://www.preventcancer.com/patients/children/ritalin.htm

3. Toxicology and Carcinogenesis Studies of Methylphenidate Hydrochloride (CAS No. 298-59-9) in F344/N Rats and B6C3F$_1$ Mice (Feed Studies), July 1995. *National Toxicology Program. Department of Health and Human Services.*
http://ntp.niehs.nih.gov/?objectid=070A08B2-F676-E37A-F6C5551ECF1D86A1

4. Medical Definitions: Jennifer R Willert, M.D., et al. *Medscape Reference.* Retrieved March 7, 2012. http://emedicine.medscape.com/article/986802-overview
http://emedicine.medscape.com/article/170205-overview

Charts and Graphs

1. Social regression and TV time for young children
2. Percentage of children watching R-rated violent movies
3. Possible contributing influences on ADHD
4. Psychotropic medication spending and use increase 1993 to 2003
5. Mental health dynamics

****

Chart 1

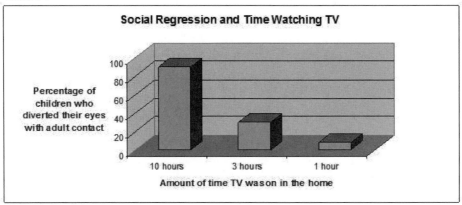

Based on study from the Japanese Pediatric Association

The Japanese Pediatric Association urges parents and doctors to keep children, especially those aged less than two, away from the television as much as possible, after research findings showed that watching too much television impaired children's ability to develop personal relationships.

Sources:

Daily Yomiuri online
http://www.yomiuri.co.jp/main//main-e.htm

Medical News Today
http://www.medicalnewstoday.com/articles/5799.php

Chart 2

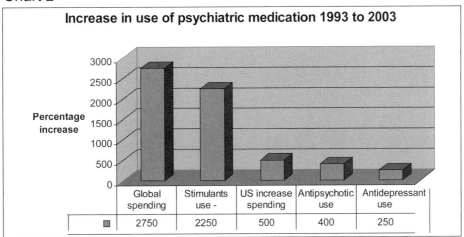

Increase in use of psychiatric medication 1993 to 2003				
Global spending	Stimulants use -	US increase spending	Antipsychotic use	Antidepressant use
2750	2250	500	400	250

Increase in stimulant use if for Australia/Britain. The statistics of this chart are primarily from the book *Rethinking ADHD*, by Ruth Neven Schmidt, et al., (as well as from other sources).

Not too be ignored is the fact that there is a lot of money to be made in the manufacturing and marketing of pharmaceutical drugs. Pharmaceutical companies are vigorous and thorough in marketing both their products, as well as their particular way of addressing mental health issues to physicians.

The result of this is that it has affected the viewpoint of the larger percentage of the medical community, including health insurance companies, who find the medical model a more cost-effective way of dealing with mental health disorders than therapy or other methods.

That combination of high profits for the pharmaceutical industry, the convenience of taking medication, rather than the difficult process of making lifestyle changes, building coping skills, and obtaining therapy when needed, as well as minimizing costs for insurance companies, has contributed to a boom in pharmaceutical spending for psychiatric drugs on all fronts, as much as has any actual increase in the rate of perceived mental health disorders.

Chart 3

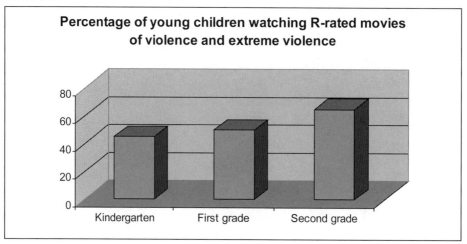

Independent survey (AYCNP), 2006, 2007, Newark, NJ, of 70 early childhood children. See *Your Child's Health,* by Barton Schmidt, M.D., F.A.A.P., about general medical guidelines and advice for parents, as well as information about possible mental and emotional repercussions for children who watch violent R-rated movies.

****

While the actual rate of children who watch violent and extremely violent R-rated movies on cable television, predominately, but also in video format, might vary from location to location, most psychology professionals would probably agree that the rate at which young children are exposed to violence in the form of violent television and movies, for children in early childhood, is an alarming trend, both for individual children and for society as a whole. In one second grade, few parents provided any guidelines or restrictions on their children, allowing the majority to regularly watch R-rated movies of extreme violence, with or without supervision.

Parents and educators should be aware that this can affect a child's emotions, their ability to demonstrate compassion, as well as a child's mental health. Further, watching violent R-rated movies can affect a child's academic performance, and children in the Bronx who did not watch violent R-rated movies, got better grades than children who did. Additionally, for some children, violent R-rated movies might contribute to some of the symptoms of ADHD in some children, and depression (especially for girls) for others.

Children and teens who demonstrate violent tendencies or have difficulties with anger in their interactions with others, might be affected emotionally from violence in the media, or demonstrating behaviors learned, over long-term exposure to violence. Sometimes movies of sadistic violence as well as violent video games are viewed on public school media equipment in after school programs or at other times. This should be a concern to principals and other administrators in public schools.

Chart 4

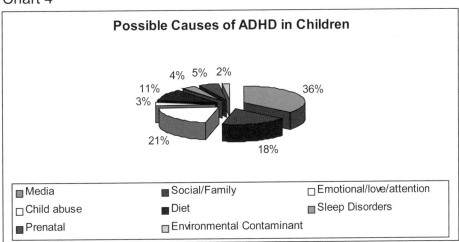

Possible Causes of ADHD in Children

4% 5% 2%
11%
3%
36%
21%
18%

■ Media	■ Social/Family	□ Emotional/love/attention
□ Child abuse	■ Diet	■ Sleep Disorders
■ Prenatal	▨ Environmental Contaminant	

This is a suggested list of possible causes or contributing influences for ADHD in children, and to a certain extent, adults. Joel Nigg, Ph.D., in his book *What Causes ADHD?,* provides evidence that there are causes for the disorder. It is not something that arises unbidden, and that while there is a genetic predisposition for ADHD, it is the combination of genetic predisposition with a number of other factors that leads to the actual disorder, in all probability.

The percentages offered in this graph are intuitive rather than scientific, and are meant to be applicable over a broad population and not for individuals. Some of the categories overlap such as Social/Family and Emotional/love/attention, child abuse. It must be remembered also, that any gaps in family life can contribute to other factors, even prenatal, in that, if a person's life is not in good order to begin with, then there is a greater chance that prenatal care might not be adequate, or that a child will not receive the love and attention he needs.

Poverty might also put one at greater risk for environmental contaminants such as lead poisoning. A larger percentage of old tenements may still have lead paint on the walls and paint chips that children might ingest. So, many of the factors in this summary may be co-dependent or mutually influenced.

Chart 5. Mental Health Dynamics Chart

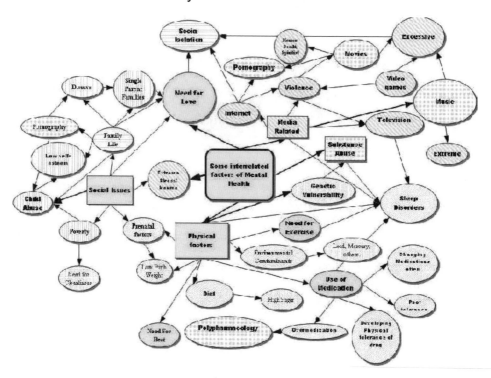

Please see webpage for larger, readable version of mental health dynamics chart
www.winmentalhealth.com/images//charts/mentalhealthchart.jpg

Professor emeritus of Vermont University and former president of the American Psychological Association (APA), George Albee, Ph.D., felt that social issues were at the root of mental health disorders for a significant percentage of the population.

Professor emeritus of Cornell University and co-founder of the *Head Start* (preschool) program in the United States, Urie Bronfenbrenner, and his Bioecological Model of mental health, provided for multiple factors, micro and macro, which contribute to mental health and mental health disorders. The mental health chart above is loosely configured around that model. Bronfenbrenner's Model for mental health is infinitely more useful than the popular medical model, on which most modern psychiatry (not psychology) is based.

Additionally, other models of mental health such as Positive Psychology, which originated and continues to flourish in Penn State University, and the similarly nuanced Strengths Model of psychology, provides a positive psychological perspective that is positive and advantageous, as opposed to the generally negative perspective of the medical model, which basically involves labeling, prescribing and coping.

Bibliography & Index

ADDA Subcommittee on ADHD Coaching. (2002, November). The ADHD Guiding Principles for Coaching Individuals with Attention Deficit Disorder. *Attention Deficit Disorder Association (ADDA).* Retrieved from www.add.org/articles /coachingguide.html

ADHD & Coexisting Conditions: Tics and Tourette Syndrome. (2005*). National Resource Center on AD/HD.* Retrieved from CHADD website http://www.help4adhd.org/documentsM/ WK5a1 .pdf

ADHD in Children. (2010). *Mayo Clinic.* Retrieved from http://www.mayoclinic.com/health/adhd/DS00275

Adult ADHD (2010). *Mayo Clinic.* Retrieved from http://www.mayoclinic.com/health/adult-adhd/DS01161

Antidepressants with Novel Mechanism of Action. (2011, November). *Virginia Commonwealth University Research.* Retrieved from http://www.research.vcu.edu/ott/licensable_technologies/flash/DUK-10-43.htm

Armstrong, T. (1997). *The Myth of the A.D.D. Child - 50 Ways to Improve Your Childs Behavior & Attention Span Without Drugs, Labels or Coercion.* New York: Penguin-Putman.

Ashley, S. Ph.D. (2005). *ADD / ADHD Answer Book - The Top 275 Questions Parents Ask.* Naperville, II: Sourcebooks, Inc.

Attention Deficit/ Attention Deficit Hyperactivity Disorder. (2011, December 12). *Center for Disease Control and Prevention. Department of Health and Human Services,* Retrieved from http://www.cdc.gov/ncbddd/adhd/research.html

Attention-deficit/hyperactivity disorder (ADHD) in children –Treatment and Drugs. (2001, February). *Mayo Clinic.* Retrieved from http://www.mayoclinic.com/health/adhd/DS00275/DSECTION=treatments-and-drugs

Barkley, R., Ph.D. (1997). *ADHD and the Nature of Self Control.* New York: Guildford.

Barkley, R., PhD., Murphy, K. R., Fischer, M. (2008). *ADHD in Adults: What the Science Says.* New York: Guildford.

Barkley, R., PhD. (1995). *Taking Charge of ADHD: The Complete, Authoritative Guide for Parents.* New York: Guilford.

Barroqueiro, D., Ed.D. (2006, May). The Art of Embracing AD/HD. *Attention Deficit Disorder Association (ADDA).* Retrieved from http://www.add.org/e-newsletters/May07.htm

Barrow, K. (2006, July 6). The Ritalin Generation Goes to College. *About.com newsletter.* Retrieved from http://www.about.com

Bee, H., Boyd., D. (2007). *The Developing Child, 11th Edition.* Boston: Pearson.

Behavior & Development: the Trouble with TV. Too much television can have a negative effect on your child's math and reading scores. (2005, November). *Parents Magazine.* Retrieved from http://www.parents com/parents/story jsp

Beyond pills: 5 conditions you can improve with lifestyle changes. *Harvard Health Newsletter.* Retrieved December 2011 from http://www.health.harvard.edu.

Bibliotherapy: Reading Your Way to Mental Health. (2007, July 31). *The Wall Street Journal.*

Blood Test Might Predict How Well a Depressed Patient Responds to Antidepressants. (2011, Dec 15). *Science Daily.* Retrieved from http://www.sciencedaily.com/releases/2011/12/111215135853.htm

Bronfenbrenner's Ecological Systems Theory. *National-Louis University.* Retrieved January, 2012 from http://pt3.nl.edu/paquetteryanwebquest.pdf.

Bruhn, K., Waltz, S., Stephani, U. (2007, March). Screen sensitivity in photosensitivity children and adolescents: patient dependent and stimulus dependent factors. *Epileptic Disorders.* Retrieved from http://www.ncbi.nlm.nih.gov/pubmed/17307713

Carey, B. (2007, May 3). FDA Expands Suicide Warnings on Drugs. *The New York Times.*

Case, C., Dalley, T. (2008). *Art Therapy with Children: From Infancy to Adolescence.* London: Karnac.

Child population: Number of children (in millions) ages 0–17 in the United States by age, 1950–2010 and projected 2030–2050. *ChildStates.gov.* Retrieved February, 2012 from http://www.childstats.gov/americaschildren/tables/pop1.asp?popup=true (Retrieved 2011, February).

Christakis, D., Zimmerman, F., DiGiussepe, D. (2004, April 4). Early Television Exposure and Subsequent Attentional Problems in Children. *Pediatrics. Vol. 113, No. 4.* Retrieved from http://pediatrics.aappublications.org/content/113/4/708.abstract

Cummings, H.M., Vandewater, E.A. (2007, July). Relation of Adolescent Video Game Play to Time Spent in Other Activities. *Archives of Pediatric and Adolescent Medicine. 161:* 684 - 689. Retrieved from http://archpedi.ama-assn.org/cgi/content/abstract/161/7/684?maxtoshow=&hits=10&RESULTFORMAT=&fulltext=cummings+gamers&searchid=1&FIRSTINDEX=0&resourcetype=HWCIT

Depression (Major Depression) - Depression and anxiety: Exercise eases symptoms. (2011, October 1). *Mayo Clinic.* Retrieved from http://www.mayoclinic.com/health/depression-and-exercise/MH00043

Dogget, M., PhD. (2004). ADHD and drug therapy: is it still a valid treatment? *School of Education, Colorado State University.* Retrieved from http://scottsdale.brainadvantage.com/PDF/ADHD%20and%20drug%20therapy.pdf

Don't let your baby watch too much TV says Japanese experts. (2004, February). *Medical News Online.* Retrieved from http://www.medicalnewstoday.com/articles/5799.php

Drug Withdrawal. (2004, December 20). *Time Magazine.* Retrieved from http://www.time. com/time/magazine/article/0,9171,1009789,00.html

Eide, B., Eide, F. (2006). *The Mislabeled Child.* New York: Hyperion.

Edwards, E. (1989). *Drawing on the Right Side of the Brain.* New York: Tarcher/Putnam.

Fartery, E. (2000, October 4). Attention Deficit Disorder and a Mom's Heartaches. *The Record.* Retrieved from http://www.web2.bccls .org/web2/tram p2.exe/see_record

FDA Alert: Liver Injury Risk and Market Withdrawal. (2005, October). Alert for Healthcare Professionals: Pemoline Tablets and Chewable Tables (marketed as Cylert). *US Food and Drug Administration, Center for Drug Evaluation and Research.* Retrieved from http://www.fda.gov/downloads/Drugs/DrugSafety/PostmarketDrugSafetyl InformationforPatientsandProviders/ucm 126462.pdf

FDA Alert: Safety Alerts for Drugs, Biologies, Medical Devices, and Dietary Supplements. (2005, September). *FDA News. Food and Drug Administration.* Retrieved from *http://www.fda.gov/Safety/MedWatch/SafetyInformation/SafetyAlertsforHumanMedicalProducts/ucm151073.htm*

FDA Issues Public health Advisory on Strattera (Atmoxetine) for Attention Deficit Disorder. (2005, September 30). *FDA News. U. S. Food and Drug Administration.* Retrieved from http://www.fda.gov/bbs/topics/NEW S/2005/NEW 01237.html

Focusing on Instruction. *Teach ADHD.* Retrieved 2011 from http://research.aboutkidshealth.ca/teachadhdAeachingadhd/chapter6

Gardener, A. (2005, July 19). Ritalin and Cancer. *HealthDay Reporter.* Retrieved from http://www.playattention.com/attention-deficit/artides/ritalin-and-cancer/

Ghaemi, N.S., MD; Shirzadi, A.A, DO; Filkowski, M., BA. (2008, September 10). Publication Bias and the Pharmaceutical Industry: The Case of Lamotrigine in Bipolar Disorder. *Medscape. 10(9):* 211. Retrieved from http://www.ncbi.nlm.nih.gov/pmc/articles/PMC2580079

Glenmullen, J. (2005). *The Antidepressant Solution.* New York: Free Press.

Glenmullen, J. (2000). *Prozac Backlash.* New York: Simon & Schuster.

Goode, E. (2003, January 1). Study finds jump in children taking psychiatric drugs. *New York Times.*

Gopfert, M., Webster, J., Seeman, M.V. (2004). *Parental psychiatric disorder: distressed parents and their families.* Cambridge: Cambridge University Press.

Gottesman, R., Ed. (1999). *Violence in America.* New York: Charles Scribner, Sons.

Gould, M S., Walsh, T.B., Munfakh, L.J. ; Kleinman, M., Duan, N., Olfson, M., Greenhill, L., Cooper, C. (September 1, 2009). Sudden Death and Use of Stimulant Medications in Youths. *American Journal of Psychiatry, VOL. 166, No. 9. 2009;166:*992-1001. 10.1176/appi.ajp.2009.09040472. Retrieved from http://ajp.psychiatryonline.org/article.aspx?articleID=101104

Green, L, Ottoson, J. (1990). *Community and Population Health, Eighth Edition.* New York, NY: McGrawHill.

Gualtieri, T.C., Johnson, L.G. (2007). Medications Do Not Necessarily Normalize Cognition in ADHD Patients. *North Carolina Neuropsychiatry Clinics, Chapel Hill and Charlotte.* Retrieved from http://www.ncneuropsych.com/research/ADD-normalize.pdf

Hallowel, E., M.D., Ratey, J. M.D. (1994*). Driven to Distraction Recognizng and Coping with Attention Deficit Disorder from Childhood Through Adulthood*. New York: Touchstone.

Harris, G. (2006, November 23). Proof is Scant on Psychiatric Drug Mix for Young. *New York Times.*

Hill, K., Ed.D. (2005). Personal Correspondence. Paterson, NJ.

Holden, C. (2004, October 26). Prozac may actually raise anxiety levels in newborn mice. *Science Now.*

How Coaching Impacts The Academic Functioning of University Students with LD and/or ADHD. (2011). *University of North Carolina.* Retrieved from http://www.unc.edu/ AHEAD_PRESENTATION_2011_UNC_CH_FINAL_000.ppt

Huxsahl. John, E., M.D. (2010). Do Food Additives Cause ADHD? *Mayo Clinic.* Retrieved from http://www.mayoclinic.com/health/adhd/AN01721

Iannelli, V. (2006, July). ADHD in the Summer. *About.com.* Retrieved from http://pediatrics.about.com/od/adhd/a/06_adhd_summer.htm

Imam, S., M.D., MPH; Sargenet, J. M.D. (2006, October 2). Association Between Television, Movie, and Video Game Exposure and School Performance. *Pediatrics.* Retrieved from http://pediatrics.aapublications.Org/cgi/content/full/118/4/e1061

It's Easier Seeing Green - ADHD curbed when kids play outdoors. (2004, March/April). *Psychology Today.* pp. 26,27.

Kelly, R. (2005, August 8). How to Quit the Cure-SSRIs. *Newsweek.*

King, S., Waschbusch, D., Pelham W., Jr, Frankland, B. W., Andrade, B. F., Jacques, S., Corkum, P. V. (2008, December 24). Social Information Processing in Elementary-School Aged Children with ADHD: Medication Effects and Comparisons with Typical Children. *Journal of Abnormal Child Psychology.* Retrieved from http://www.springerlink .com/content/pp7675p0777q>g15/

King, W. (2007, May 8). Babies, Toddlers watch lots of TV, new study finds. *Seattle Times.* Retrieved from http://www.seatletimes.nwsource.com.

Kluger, J. (2003, November 3). Are We Giving Our Kids Too Many Drugs? *Time Magazine.*

Kuo, F., E., Taylor, A. F. (2004). A Potential Natural Treatment for Attention-Deficit/Hyperactivity Disorder: Evidence From a National Study. *American Journal of Public Health.* Retrieved from http://ajph.aphapublications.org/cgi/content/abstract/9479/1580 http://www.ncbi.nlm.nih.gov/pmc/articles/PMC1448497/

Lambert, C. (2000, May/June). The Downsides of Prozac. *Harvard Magazine.* Retrieved from http://harvardmagazine.com/2000/05/the-downsides-of-prozac.html

Lipkin, P.H., Butz, A.M., Cozen, M.A. (2003). High Dose Methylphenidate treatment of ADHD in a Preschooler. *Journal of Child and Adolescent Psychopharmacology.* Retrieved from http://www.ncbi.nlm.nih.gov/pubmed/12804131 ?dopt=Abs tract.

Literacy. (2002). *Wisconsin Department of Public Instruction.* Retrieved from *http://dpi.wi.gov/pld/pdf/sn09.pdf*

Louv, R. (2008). *Last Child in the Woods, Saving Our Children from Nature-Deficit Disorder.* Chapel Hill, NC: Algonquin Books

Lugara, J. (2004, October). Disconnected from the real world: Is the new age of media & technology killing our kid's childhoods? *Metro Parent Guide.*

Many NIH-Funded Clinical Trials Go Unpublished Over Two Years After Completion, U.S. Study Shows. (2012, January 3). *Science Daily.* Retrieved from http://www.sciencedaily.com/releases/2012/01/120103211056.htm

Marsa, L. (2005, January 5). The Prozac Paradox Why antidepressants may exacerbate depression and anxiety in some kids and teens. *Popular Science.* Retrieved from http://psychrights.org/articles/PopularScienceProzacParadoxhtm

Mate, G. (1999). *Scattered: How Attention Deficit Disorder Originates And What You Can Do About It.* New York: The Penguin Group.

McNuff, J. (2005). Personal communication. Paterson, NJ.

Medicated Child, The. (2008, January 8). *Frontline, PBS.* Retrieved from http://www.pbs.org/wgbh/pages/frontline/medicatedchild

Medicating Kids: Interview with Russell Barkley. *Frontline, PBS.* Retrieved 2008 from http://www.pbs.org/wgbh/pages/frontline/shows/medicating/interviews/barkley.html

Meijer, W. E., PhD, Heerdink, E. R., PhD, Nolen, W. A., MD, PhD, Herings, R. M. C., PhD, Leufkens, H. G. M., PhD, Egberts, A. C. G., PhD. (2004). Association of Risk of Abnormal Bleeding With Degree of Serotonin Reuptake Inhibition by Antidepressants. *Arch Intern Med. 2004;164:*2367-2370. Retrieved from http://archinte.ama-assn.org/cgi/content/full/164/21/2367?maxtoshow=&hits=10&RESULTFORMAT=&fulltext=Welmoed+E.+E.+Meijer%2C+PhD&searchid=1&FIRSTINDEX=0&resourcetype=HWCIT

Mind Launches Green agenda for Mental Health. Ecotherapy vs. retail therapy. (2007). *Heliq.* Retrieved from http://www.huliq.com/21526/mind-launches-new-green-agenda-for-mental-health

Moody, S. (2007, April 15). Jefferson Award Presented to Dan Woldow— San Francisco Schools are kissing junk food goodbye. Here's Why. *San Francisco Chronicle.* Retrieved from http://www.sfgate.com

Moore, D., T., Ph.D. (2001). *Behavioral Interventions for ADHD. Your Family Clinic.* http://www.yourfamilyclinic.com/shareware/addbehavior.html

Movig, K.L., PhD, Janssen, M.W., M.D., Jan de Waal M., MD, PhD, Kabel,P. J., MD, PhD, Leufkens, H.G.M., PhD, Egberts, A.C.G., PhD. (2003, October 27). Relationship of Serotonergic Antidepressants and Need for Blood Transfusion in Orthopedic Surgical Patients. *Archives of Internal Medicine, 203; 163*:2354-2358. Retrieved from http://www.ncbi.nlm.nih.gov/pubmed/14581256

Neven, R. Anderson, V. Godber, T. (1997). *Rethinking ADHD: Integrated approaches to helping children at home and at school.* Australia: Allen & Unwin.

Newcomb, J., M.D., Sutton, V.K., Ph.D., Zhang, S., M.S., Wilens, T., M.D., Kratochvil, C., M.D., Graham J. Emslie, G.J., M.D., D'souza, D.N., Ph.D., Schuh, L.M., M.B.A., Ph.D.,Albert J. Allen, M.D., Ph.D. (2009, August). Characteristics of Placebo Responders in Pediatric Clinical Trials of Attention-Deficit/Hyperactivity Disorder. *Journal of the American Academy of Child and Adolescent Psychiatry.* Retrieved from http://www.jaacap.com/article/S0890-8567(09)66072-X/abstract

New Jersey Teaching Notes. (2005-2012). *Association for Youth, Children and Natural Psychology (AYCNP).*

New Prozac Blues. (2004, Dec 17). *Time Magazine.* Retrieved from http://www.time.com/time/magazine/article/0,9171,1009635,00. html

Nigg, J. (2006). *What Causes ADHD? Understanding What Goes Wrong and Why.* New York: The Guilford Press

Oflaz, F., PhD, Hatipolu, S., PhD, Aydin, H., MD. (2008, March). Effectiveness of psychoeducation intervention on post-traumatic stress disorder and coping styles of earthquake survivors. *Journal of Clinical Nursing, Vol 17, Issue 5.* Retrieved from http://www.ncbi.nlm.nih.gov/pubmed/18279300

Olfman, S., (Ed). (2007). *Bipolar Children, (Childhood in America).* Westport, CT: Praeger.

Olfman, S., (Ed). (2006). *No Child Left Different, (Childhood in America).* Westport, CT: Praeger.

Olfman, S. (Ed). (2008). *The Sexualization of Childhood (Childhood in America).* Westport, CT: Praeger.

Párraga H.C, Párraga M.I, Harris D.K. (2007). Tic exacerbation and precipitation during atomoxetine treatment in two children with attention-deficit hyperactivity disorder. *Internal Journal of Psychiatry in Medicine. 37(4):*415-24.

Pearce, J. (2008, March 3). Peter Neaubauer, 94, Noted child Psychiatrist. *New York Times.* http://www.nytimes.com/2008/03/03/nyregion/03neubauer.html

Pelsser LM, Frankena K, Toorman J, Savelkoul HF, Pereir, RR, Buitelaar JK. (January 2009). A randomised controlled trial into the effects of food on ADHD.. *European Journal of Child and Adolescent Psychiatry.* http://www.ncbi.nlm.nih.gov/pubmed/18431534

Rabiner, D. (2010, March). One Reason why Children with ADHD Should be Reevaluated Each Year. *Attention Research Update.*

Rabiner D. (2006, January). Side effects rates for medications. *Attention Research Update.* Retrieved from http://www.helpforadd.com/2006/january.htm

Rabiner, D. (2006, January). Understanding Parents' Concerns about Medication Treatment. *Attention Research Update.* Retrieved from http://www.helpforadd.com/2006/january.htm

Rabiner, D. (2006). What is ADHD? *Attention Research Update* . Retrieved from http://www.helpforadd.com/what-is-adhd

Range, L. Children's Health. *Attention! For families and Adults with Attention Deficit/Hyperactivity Disorder. CHADD.*

Ratey, J. An Update on Medications used in the Treatment of Attention Deficit Disorder. *Attention Deficit Disorder Association (ADDA).* Retrieved 2005 from www.add.org.

Read for Emotional Relief. (2006). *Healthy Person.* Retrieved from http://www.healthy-person. blogspot.com/2006/11/read-for-emotional-relief.html .

Remembering George Albee. (2006). *Society for Community Research and Action.* Retrieved from http://www.scra27.org/George%20Albee.html

Richardson, W. (2005). ADHD and Stimulant Medication Abuse. *Attention Deficit Disorder Association (ADDA).* Retrieved from *http://*www.add.org/articles/med_abuse.html

Rief, S. F. (1993). *How to Reach and Teach ADD/ADHD Children.* Hoboken, NJ: Wiley & Sons.

Ritalin and Depression. (2007, March 8). *Med TV.* Retrieved from http://adhd.emedtv.com/ritalin/ritalin-and-depression.htm

Robertson, J. (1998). *Natural Prozac.* San Francisco: HarperSanFrancisco.

Rupin, T. MD, Garrison, M. PhD, Christakis, MD, MPH. (2006, November 5). A Systematic Review for the Effects of Television Viewing by Infants and Preschoolers. *Pediatrics,* pp.2025-2031.

Ryals, T, F., M.D. Retrieved April 9, 2011 from http://www.thadryals.com.

Sachs, G. (2007, March 28). Adding antidepressants to mood-stabilizing drugs does not affect (positively) bipolar depression (disorder.) study. *New England Journal of Medicine.* Retrieved from *http://www.nejm.org/doi/full/10.1056/NEJMoa064135*

Sigman, A., PhD. (2005). *Remotely Controlled: How television is damaging our lives - and what we can do about it.* London: Vermillion.

Study Shows School Breakfast Program Works in Newark. (2010, February). *Essex News.* p.9.

Schmidt, B., D. (1991). *Your Child's Health.* New York: Bantam.

Shannon, S.M., M.D.; Heckman. E. (2007). *Please Don't Label My Child: Break the Doctor-Diagnosis-Drug Cycle and Discover Safe, Effective Choices for Your Child's Emotional Health.* Ammaus, PA: Rodale.

Side Effects. *Rx.com.* Retrieved 2008 from https://ecom.nhin.com/nhin/servlet/DrugSearchEntry?CHAIN_ID=119080

Study finds early Ritalin exposure may have long term effects. (2004, December 20). *Mental Health Weekly.* Retrieved from http://www3.interscience.wiley.com

Szabo, L. (2006, March 27). ADHD Treatment is Getting a Workout; Doctors Turn to Exercise, other Drug Alternatives. *USA Today.* Retrieved from http://www.usatoday.com

Timmes, A. (2005). ADHD Through the Eyes of Girls. *NJ County Family Magazine.*

Tips to help live with ADD. *Living with ADD.* Retrieved 2006 from http://www.livingwithADD.com/tips.html

Walker, S. (1998). *The Hyperactivity Hoax.* New York: St. Martin's Press.

Wallis, C. (2006, March 19). The Multitasking Generation. *Time Magazine,* Retrieved from http://www.time.com/time/magazine/article/0,9171,1174696,00.html

Waschbusch, D.A., PhD, Pelham, W. E., Jr., PhD, Waxmonsky, J., MD, Johnston, C., PhD. (2009). Are There Placebo Effects in the Medication Treatment of Children With Attention-Deficit Hyperactivity Disorder*? Journal of Developmental & Behavioral Pediatric.* Retrieved from http://www.cogsci.ucsd.edu/~mboyle/COGS11-Summer/COGS11-website/presentation%20papers/placebos-adhd-effects.pdf

What are the real risks of antidepressants? (2005, May). *Harvard Health.* Retrieved from http://www.health.harvard.edu/newsweek/What_are_the_real_risks_of_antidepressants.htm

What is ADHD? *Kids Health.* Retrieved August 14, 2009 from http://kidshealth.org/parent/medical/learning/adhd.html

Wilens, T. (2006, January). Multisite controlled study of OROS methylphenidate in the treatment of adolescents with Attention-Deficit/Hyperactivity Disorder. *Archives of Pediatric and Adolescent Medicine. 148(8),* 859-861. Retrieved from http://archpedi.ama-assn.org/cgi/content/full/160/1/82

Wilens, T. E., Faraone, S. V., Biederman, J., Gunawardene, S. (2003). Does Stimulant Therapy Of Attention-Deficit Hyperactivity Disorder Beget Later Substance Abuse A Meta-Analytic Review Of The Literature. *Pediatrics, 111 179 185.* Retrieved from http://pediatrics.aappublications.0rg/cgi/content/abstract/111/1/179

Williams, J., Zickler, P. (2003, June). Researchers Probe for Clues to ADHD Medications' Protective Effects. *National Institute on Drug Abuse.* Retrieved from http://archives.drugabuse.gov/NIDA_Notes/NNVol18N1/Researchers.html

Wdraich, M. L, M.D., Wilson, D. B., Ph.D, White, W., M.D. (1995). The Effect of Sugar on Behavior or Cognition in Children. A Meta-analysis. *JAMA. 274(20);*1616-1621. Retrieved from http://jama.ama-assn.org/cgi/content/abstract/274/20/1617

Yatko, M.D. (2012). *Trancework.* New York: Routledge.

Young, J, Giwerc, D. (2005). Just What is Coaching*? Attention Deficit Disorder Association (ADDA).* Retrieved from http://www.add.org.

Zimmerman, M., M.D., Ruggero, C, Ph.D., Chelminski, Ph.D., Young, D., Ph.D. (2007, December 24). Is Bipolar Disorder Overdiagnosed? *The Journal of Clinical Psychiatry* Retrieved from http://www.psychiatrist.com/abstracts/abstracts.asp?abstract=200806/060808.htm

Index

114